WHERE DOES THE FIGHT COME FROM?

HOW I SURVIVED CHILDHOOD CANCER

DR. BRADLEY SCHMIDT

WHERE DOES THE FIGHT COME FROM?
How I Survived Childhood Cancer

A memoir by
Dr. Bradley Schmidt

ISLAND ONE PUBLISHING
MARIETTA, GEORGIA

<u>WHERE DOES THE FIGHT COME FROM?</u>
How I Survived Childhood Cancer

Published by:
Island One Publishing, LLC
P.O. Box 71092
Marietta, Georgia 30007

ISBN: 978-0-615-59246-6

First Printing: February 2012
Printed in the United States of America

To the best of my knowledge, this story is factual and is supported by documentation, interviews, and photos. Some of the names have been changed due to respect, or lack of permission.

Additional Copies of this book may be purchased at
www.drbradschmidt.com

Cover design by Dr. Bradley D. Schmidt. Cover layout designed by Kimberly Martin of Jera Publishing.

Dedication

This book is dedicated with love and admiration to my parents ~ Charles and Jackie Schmidt

<u>About the Author</u>

Dr. Brad Schmidt Is a childhood cancer survivor. He has fought a life-long battle with the after effects of surviving Neuroblastoma, including (3) invasive surgeries, the development of Scoliosis, leg and spinal bracing, and deficiencies in walking. As a baby, he was dealt a tremendous setback when the aftermath of his (3) surgeries left him unable to stand or even begin to walk. The doctors had informed his parents that he would at best be in a wheelchair for the rest of his life.

Through a remarkable innate drive and perseverance, he not only survived the operations and procedures that threatened his life, he later developed the ability to crawl, stand, and then walk of his own power. The aftermath of the fight with cancer, radiation, chemotherapy, and learning to walk were only the beginning of his challenges. As a young boy, he developed a case of scoliosis of the spine as a side effect of his surgeries. With this deformity came another set of circumstances. The scoliosis left him moderately handicapped and a shorter left leg with limited use.

Against the advice of the doctors, at the age of 10, Brad started hitting a racquetball around a court with his father in order to get some form of exercise. He started playing racquetball initially with his scoliosis brace on, and later shed to brace in order to pursue the sport. As he matured into adulthood, he became a state and nationally ranked player. With the doctors initially informing his parents that he may not even survive the surgeries and therapies to eradicate the Neuroblastoma, Brad has survived the odds and endured the challenges as a handicapped individual.

With his intention to help people, Brad went on to college and to graduate school. He attended college in Atlanta, Georgia; and later graduated as a Doctor of Chiropractic in 1999. He currently resides in Marietta, Georgia with his wife, Allison. His presence is still prominent in racquetball today as he travels around the southeast region on the United States competing tournaments and promoting the sport that gave him his mobility and life. He is self-employed, now working with several law firms as an Accident Investigator, consulting in the assessment of personal injury clients.

Dr. Brad, with his desire to assist people with health challenges and situations, is developing a program in the form of motivational materials, speaking engagements, and internet sources in order to share his tremendous and uplifting story.

Table of Contents

You gain strength and confidence by every experience in which you really stop and look fear in the face. You are able to say to yourself, 'I lived through this horror. I can take the next thing that comes along'. ....You must do the thing you think you cannot do."

~ Eleanor Roosevelt

INTRODUCTION

All that we are inundated with is the menagerie of negative stories in the media about the struggles of the human condition and the quest to prevail and exist on planet earth. We are informed daily of the horrific, sensational stories of crime, murder, war and natural disasters. These stories are meant to target our emotions, capture our attention, and pose on us the question of our own mortality. People absorb these stories, and I believe, by doing so, adversely affect their collective unconsciousness.

Continued and repetitive, negative news about the human condition works against us all. Very seldom do you hear a story, which in itself has a positive, lasting component that dials into us. This concept of a positive story in the media lacks the impact of a negative one mainly for the shock value. The negative, dramatic, and over-powering stories are the mainstay of our society.

This mainstay takes the drive out of ones desire to succeed in his or her way or fashion. Life is defiantly a struggle; no matter what country, group, family, region, socioeconomic class one is from. Ideally, we are to be born with all the living components that nature has designed us to have. On a natural level, we are born into this world naked, with an undeveloped brain, the necessary senses, arms and legs, and innate guidance system which will aid us in our quest to grow and prosper to ensure that we live a long life.

But what if you are born at a disadvantage; I mean a disadvantage that has a grip on you before society can impose its own guidance system. What does it take to have the power to overcome and master that disadvantage? Or, even better, to take that disadvantage, and some how turn it into a purpose, a reason, and an advantage for that individual. This book is about my life. It is a chronological story of my struggle to make it to adulthood and further succeed in life after being dealt a tremendous challenge at birth. It is a story of my triumph.

I was born with a type of cancer called Neuroblastoma. This type of cancer had a potential to end my life soon after birth. Through many medical procedures and an innate drive to survive, I am alive and thriving. I am a product of my environment; the end result of a *gift* that I now realize that I was given early in life. The purpose of telling my story is to pass on my experiences to others in the hope of showing people how the human body has the innate capacity and ability to overcome any adversity…or in my case, turn an adversity into a life long celebra-tion…..This is my story.

INTRODUCTION

"Don't tell people how to live their lives....Just tell them stories; they will figure it out for themselves"

~ Randy Pausch

CHAPTER 1:
Cancer

When people hear the word cancer in this day an age; they think the worst. The "C" word is a death sentence unless it is caught early enough in ones life. It is a requirement that we all do screenings – breast, ovarian, testicular, skin, throughout our lives in order to detect cancer early enough to catch the cancer in its least invasive expression. I find it amazing of the vast numbers of types of cancer prevalent in society today. I ask myself...'Where did all these cancer cases come from?' 'Why are certain cancers more glamorized in the media when a celebrity sheds a demand for awareness?' 'Why do only the main types of cancers get most of the focus?' It seems that there are more questions than answers.

What if the type of cancer was undetectable and hidden until it was a monster? What if *you* were dealt cancer with the gift of just being born? No prescreening test could gage and measure the amount, type, or invasiveness at that point. This was a card I was dealt when I came into this world. I was born with a type of cancer called *Neuroblastoma*. This a tumor-like presentation cancer located in the neural ganglia of its host. Basically, it is a nerve cancer. It was later determined that my cancer had already taken hold of me inside the womb.

This whole endeavor of constructing my story to share with the world started when my mother told me she wanted to give me a box of baby items and records. I said, "records from what?" It turns out it was my medical records from many key points in my life. I brought them back to my home where they sat in my office in a corner under a desk for some weeks. One morning, I decided to go through the box as I was doing a little cleaning. I broke into this box and began to unpack all these miscellaneous medical records. I was unaware at the time, that I was going back and unraveling the interconnected details of a journey that comprised my life.

I spread them out in the middle of my office. It was not until I sat there and began to read and arrange these old yellowing files in some sort of chronological order; that something came about me. I read each document and looked at dates and signatures. I read all the paragraphs, all the procedures and different prognosis statements written by the numerous doctors. I read everything with a great understanding; I knew what all the medical terms meant due to my education.

It was so interesting for me to go back in time that day.....I spent the rest of the afternoon and early evening on the floor with all this historical paperwork surrounding me like I was sitting on a paper island. My eyes began to well up with tears as many memories were stirred up from the basement of my mind. It is a powerful thing for a person to shed light on a painful and difficult past. Many of my difficult childhood experiences I had mentally placed in a downstairs room of my mind. These memories were like a huge ominous storm that was pushed out to sea; unable to rein it's fury on land. My reality was to keep my early experiences hidden away as if to be forgotten. Many memories both traumatic and enjoyable are never forgotten; they just need a little assistance to bring light to them.

I had basically forgotten much of the earliest memories of my battles with cancer and the aftermath. Up until this time, I liked it that way. If you mentally block off memories, over time, it is as if they did not happen. Along with all of this business of forgetting the past, I also struggled with being perceived as physically "normal". I just wanted to blend into the population. I did not want to be treated any different or given any special privileges; and I protected this position on this matter, as it has been the most important focus of my life.

After breaking into and organizing the contents of the box, I had an awakening. It was an awakening in the sense that I realized that all the old and decaying papers in the box were the pieces and clues to the events of my life. It was on that day that I decided to change the way I look at my past. The papers that surrounded me on the floor of the room documented the events and milestones that make up the fabric of who I have become as an adult.

I could not have made it to this day if all the events of my life did not occur in *exactly* the way they did. After reading the box of records, going through the events and thoughts in my mind that day, I just began to reflect. I felt like I was a solitary man walking down a long, empty hallway lined with doors on both sides. I have always had forward momentum in my life. I seldom stopped, and mentally looked back at all the doors I have opened and closed along my journey that is my life. I have *always* looked forward. It was as if I had been through a powerful and ominous thunderstorm. I made it from one end of the storm to another; pounded by the rain, but never hit by the lightening.

We have all experienced bad storms from time to time. When we make it through bad weather we tend to look at it in a different way. Maybe we look at them with a special respect. Large thunderstorms are beautiful when you see them forming, or you have driven through and can look back at them. It was at that point of stopping and looking back that I realized I have been on an amazing journey. The trials and tribulations of how I fought and overcame are the foundation that defines who I have become.

Cancer is a permanent fixture today in the news. We are given updates on the "battle with cancer" like a World

CHAPTER 1: Cancer

War II updates in the newsreels of the 1940's. The media machine tells us all the types we are fighting, where they come from, and the statistics that we as the human race have to overcome. As I did my research for this book, it became apparent to me that the types of cancer, and what I call *"the cancer machine"* has become larger and more prevalent. Cancer has become a rather big business. The fear that is associated and generated when we hear the word cancer is troubling to me. I reside in Atlanta, Georgia, where many of my treatments and surgeries took place. As I drive throughout Atlanta, I see the billboards and the advertisements for the various clinics and hospitals that all claim to be "specialist" in the battle against cancer. I even hear all the advertisements on the radio as well. All of these advertisements and messages are mixed in with the car ads, retail sales ads, and concert and sporting events; these are the main staple of messages that the media wants us to hear and see.

In my opinion, the media is informing us that... not 'if' we get cancer, but '**when**' we get cancer...and we all will get at some point. When have a strange symptom or a negative result on a screening test, we need to seek out this or that specialty group. This specialty group will treat you in the most "effective" way; with a "state of the art" medical approach; to get you back on track, and on with your life. One interesting fact that I discovered while doing research for this book; there are more people who make a living off of cancer than people who actually have cancer. It has evolved into a rather large economy. It seems to me that these clinics just come right out and say it these days through their advertisements; cancer=fear. They say it in a way that dials in on our emotions. We continually are reinforced with this message. If you hear it enough, over and over again, people tend to believe it. Using fear has become the primary emotion elicited when cancer is mentioned.

In doing statistical analysis of the current state of cancer, the numbers are over whelming. According to the a report published in Dec 7th 2009 in the journal <u>Cancer</u>, over all cancer rates in new cases have declined. After researching the information it became apparent to me that the number of cases are staying somewhat constant, only the frequency and types of cases seem to change. Men and women have different challenges in regards to the numerous presentations that cancer manifests itself. Most of the cancers cases on the forefront of the news are situations that come about by exposure to certain environments, a side effect of the ingestion of some food or use of products, or even the use or exposure to situations where we are informed that the outcome will surely guarantee an experience with cancer.

Most of the more deadly, fast acting cancers show up after being in disguise, like a demon hidden in the body somewhere, only to show itself after it is too late to begin to treat it. The medical community now has a very good idea, through statistics, how long we will live when and if we are diagnosed with any one of the many different cancer presentations. The cancer experience has even been organized into levels of aggressiveness, each of which has their own timeline on accordance to our age and gender. All of this is depended on the medical approach in handling a treatment plan, and not to mention, the financial capabilities of the patient. I ask myself, where are all these cancer types coming from? 30 years ago, it appeared there were only a handful of types of cancer, and prevalence of cases. When you were diagnosed with cancer in the 1950's and 60's, you went to a small, undisclosed section of a hospital to deal with the situation. Today, the story is quite different. Cancer has become one of the leading causes of death in America.

We now have large medical facilities in major cities all over the United States and the world that our so specialized in dealing with cancer that you may have to move to a different city just to take on the battle. The size of the global economy of dealing with cancer is immense. To this day, I still am quiet overwhelmed, and amazed that I made it through all the procedures and treatments in dealing with my health and well being. My respect for the medical personnel, which saved my life, is grounded in that emotion.

I do have the uttermost admiration for the medical community in regards to cancer. Many amazing breakthroughs and triumphs have taken place just in the last decade alone have occurred to decrease the numbers of new cases. I just disagree on the approach taken to inform, treat, and educate the people about the topic of cancer. Fear is used as a tool in many different arenas to control people and make them conform or else something bad may happen. Throughout history, this fear emotion has been tapped into on many different levels. It is used in war; governments use it on their populations, corporations use it on us in advertising. We hear this in flu shot advertisements, ecoli reports, and cancer pre-screening campaigns. I am just against using fear as a way to approach a conflict. I feel that one party is trying to control another with an agenda not beneficial to the group being controlled. In my opinion, just using a fear-based mentality in regards to medical conditions has placed us at a tremendous disadvantage in our quest to battle and treat this demonic threat.

CHAPTER 2:
NEUROBLASTOMA AND SURGERY

Cancer appears in the body in a variety of forms, states of aggressiveness, basically a plethora of presentations. My cancer was in the form of a tumor called Neuroblastoma, which located itself next to my left lower spine. This tumor had already begun to develop while I was inside my mother's womb. To this day, Neuroblastoma is considered a rare type of childhood cancer. Most of the cases that are reported occur in children under five years of age. Neuroblastoma is a cancer of specialized nerve cells, called neural crest cells. These cells are involved in the development of the nervous system and other tissues. This type of cancer can occur anywhere in the body, but it is most often in one of the adrenal glands in the abdomen. The adrenal glands are specialized glands, which are found above the kidneys. They release hormones to maintain blood pressure, and enable us to respond to stress. In some children, as was the case with me, the Neuroblastoma can occur in nerve tissue alongside the spinal cord in the neck, chest, abdomen, or pelvis. The ideology or cause of Neuroblastoma is unknown to this day. Like other cancers, it is not infectious and cannot be passed.

WHERE DOES THE FIGHT COME FROM?

In the medical arena today, Neuroblastoma is classified in several stages form 1 to 4s; from localized to a localized tumor with spreading to other vital areas of the body; basically just stages of aggressiveness. However, all the stages are risky and warrant concern. When a child is diagnosed, the path of medical treatment is surgery, depending on the position of the tumor. Following surgery, the child will have to endure near toxic levels of chemotherapy. And lastly as a follow up to ensure that all the cancer has been removed, radiation therapy. Typically, the child is unable to survive the path of treatment. The trauma and threat to the body is immense. This is why the survival rates are so low even in 2012.

Because my battle with cancer started before I came into this world; it had plenty of time to develop before it was accurately diagnosed. I was born in the late 1960's in Fullerton, California. My parents, Charles and Jackie Schmidt were basking in the glory of bringing their fourth baby boy into the world. My mother later informed me that they were wishing for a girl but were very happy with a boy. According to my records and my interviews with my family members, I was a perfect baby boy. I showed no clinical manifestations of any kind for the first few months of life.

My parents, my three brothers, and myself were then relocated 2 months after I was born, to Atlanta, Georgia due to a new job that was awaiting my father. My first few months of life were a "complete joy" my mother later told me. I was progressing and adapting to life as a newborn as we as a family relocated to Atlanta. It was not until October 1968 that everything changed. My oldest brother was holding me one day and brought to my mothers attention that the lower left area of my back appeared swollen and felt hard to the touch. I was too young to show any signs of crawling yet; but my mother thought it was a tight muscle. My parents thought it might be a muscle pull or something of that nature. With concern, they made an appointment with my new doctor in Atlanta, Dr. Michael Levine. Upon examination by Dr Levine, with his great compassion and concern that my parents later told me he exemplified; referred my case to Dr. Gerald T Zwiren, M.D.

Dr. Zwiren examined me at the end of January 1969; and in a letter dated January 31, 1969 back to Dr. Levine, Dr. Zwiren stated that he had discovered a "mass" in my lower left lumbar area; probably a lipoma and possibly a tumor. He informed Dr. Levine that he had scheduled "little Bradley" to be admitted to Egleston Hospital for excision of this mass on February 7th, 1969.

On February 7th, 1969, at the age of 5 months, I had my first operation to remove a mass from my lower spinal region. The pathology report later confirmed that the diagnosis was Neuroblastoma. According to the operative report, Dr. Zwiren removed a portion of the tumor via an incision through my lower left spinal region. Most of the mass was removed during this initial operation. According to the report, I tolerated the procedure well. After removing only a portion of the tumor, I was then subjected to treatment with intravenous Cytoxan and radiation therapy. My next surgery was scheduled for February 17th, 1969 to remove the rest of the mass. My parents were devastated. My father fainted and fell to the floor upon hearing all this news while meeting with Dr. Zwiren. I have to step outside of this story for a moment. It must have been almost unbearable for my parents to handle this situation. The common denominator for all parents of every newborn that comes into this world is to relish, celebrate, and cherish the experience. The mental pain and torture of the threat of loosing a newborn either through a medical disorder or by accident; just must be almost unfathomable. Looking back on my life, I would have to say that the heroic efforts of my parents during this period of my life have become their most honored attributes for me.

My parents knew nothing about this type of cancer, and how could this happen to their newborn? They were informed that next invasive surgery could possibly end my life. Dr. Zwiren told them that it was so important to get as much of the tumor removed if there would be any chance of survival; therefore a second surgery was crucial.

My second surgery consisted of going through my abdomen to excise the rest of the tumor. The question was if a baby could handle such an operation so invasive after just having surgery ten days prior. The operative report for the second surgery to remove the rest of the tumor via an incision through my abdomen reads like a dissection report of an autopsy. Most of my organs and intestines were displaced, along with the separation of many muscle groups just to get at the rest of the Neuroblastoma growing next to my spine. A large percentage of the growth was removed; a small section of the tumor was left untouched due to its location next to my spine. Abbreviated cuts were completed to related muscle groups as well as the full removal of my left Psoas muscle. The Psoas muscle is involved in the lumbar spine and hip movement associated with flexion of the hip. Also, with the invasive surgery, my nerves to my left quadriceps muscle group had to be compromised in order to remove the tumor. The postoperative report stated the tumor was about 7cms x 7cms in size and showing signs of still growing. In relation to the body size of a baby, 7cms is large. I also had most of my para-spinal muscles removed with the invasiveness of the procedures. This group of muscles is located next to the spine in the low back region or lumbar region.

WHERE DOES THE FIGHT COME FROM?

At some point early in April of 1969, after receiving massive doses of radiation and chemotherapy to annihilate the rest of the tumor; I had a third surgery. This consisted of going through my previous abdominal incision to investigate the site of the tumor. With this surgery, Dr. Zwiren could see what remained of the Neuroblastoma was only a small area of scar tissue. Basically the tumor was destroyed. With my third surgery completed, I was stitched up and was transported to intensive care to recover. My parents and family were very grateful by this time. My parents told me they took turns coming down to the hospital to be with me and watch my monitors. Dr. Zwiren later told in an interview I had with him in 1989; he honestly did not think I would make it through the second surgery. He stated it was such a risky and invasive operation for a baby to endure. He said he felt bad that he informed my parents that I could die from the surgery alone, but it was the only option; the tumor must be removed. When Dr. Zwiren returned to the hospital the following morning, he went immediately to intensive care to see me. "Your little heart monitor was still going....just amazing". He would later tell me, "You were just a little fighter".

It was a few days later that while in recovery, my whole body began to swell and turn red. I also had a fever at the same time. I developed septicemia, a blood infection, during this recovery. I was placed in isolation in order to facilitate recovery. It was later determined that my stitches from third operation had somehow became infected. It took a few weeks to get to a point in my recovery where I could go home.

The aftermath of the first months of my life had taken a toll on my body before I could even begin to crawl; *but I was alive.* With all that was done to save my life, my parents were informed that I might never have the ability to walk. Many of the support muscle groups of the pelvis and lower left lumbar regions were removed to excise the tumor; *but I was alive.* At any time later on down the road, cancer may present someplace else in my body; *but I was alive.* This was the cost of doing all these procedures and my parents understood this.

My mother told me this whole ordeal had taken a tremendous emotional and physical toll on her and my father. They later told me they do not know how they made it through that difficult time with working, raising 3 other boys, and covering all the bases as my father put it. They just wanted me home to complete their family and get back to some type of normalcy. After I recovered from the septicemia and was somewhat stable with the removal of my stitches, I was released form Egleston Hospital and sent home to begin a long journey of guarded recovery.

CHAPTER 3:
ROAD TO RECOVERY

By the age of one, I had endured so much. For the next year and a half my parents and brothers spent time with me helping me recover from this experience. Even though I was very young to remember this specific period of my life, I can only imagine that it must have been a difficult experience for my family. When interviewing my parents about this time in my life, to this day their eyes well up with tears when trying to describe what it was like to see your youngest child, struggling to get through a day. This period in time also consisted of endless doctor appointments to make sure that I was healing properly.

It was shortly after the age of one that I showed signs of attempting to crawl. My parents said, as I would try to crawl, I would drag my weaker left leg. The neurological innervation package or circuit had been intersected and clipped just to extract as much of the Neuroblastoma as possible. The left Psoas muscle was removed during surgery as well. The Psoas muscle is a major supporter of the pelvis and lower spine. My parents recalled that they were informed after the second surgery that by doing this possibly compromised my ability to ever walk. At best, I would be in a wheelchair, or be able to be mobile with the assistance of a leg brace.

This possible inability to ever walk was the cost of saving my life; this was how my father told me they took this news. I was now on a path of healing and recovery. As I progressed, I crawled more and more; "dragging my leg around" as my mother put it. I would crawl up on furniture by the age of two. Holding myself up with furniture helped me become more stable in my movements.

It was about this time that I began to show signs of developing scoliosis of the spine. All of the para-spinal muscles had been removed on the left side of my low back to excise the tumor. This set up a situation where the strong para-spinal muscles along with other muscle groups of the pelvis and spine began "pulling" to the strong side when growth started. By doing so, starts a process where the spine becomes unstable and curved which leads to vertebral growth plate deformities. So needless to say, scoliosis became the chief concern as I physically matured.

By the age of three, I was back to the specialists to get fitted for a special brace called a Milwaukee Scoliosis Brace and a left leg brace. The Milwaukee Brace consisted of a plastic pelvic girdle with a bar in the front and two bars in the back extending up to my neck. They were attached to a metal ring around my neck with hard pads that supported the base of my skull. There were hard pads and leather straps on the upper and lower sections of this apparatus. As I stated earlier in this book, the brace looked like a medieval torture device.

Its main purpose was to support and immobilize the spine in hopes of preventing the curvature from increasing. This type of brace had to constantly be adjusted in order to work effectively. Each of the bars had holes where different adjustments could be manipulated in order to put reverse pressure on the spine. This type of brace had to be re-manufactured as the body of the patient grew. At the time, this type of brace was state-the-art, seen as the only way of effectively dealing with advancing scoliosis.

While wearing this Milwaukee brace for up to 20 hours a day, I was required to also wear a support brace on my entire left leg. My recollection of this whole endeavor started for me at about the age of 3. I recall wearing both the leg brace and the scoliosis around our home in Atlanta, Georgia. As I began to stand up with the support of the furniture in our living room, basically using the furniture to walk around upright. I started to take the leg brace off by pulling on the straps. My mother said I was trying to walk without the leg brace. With my return to the orthopedics office, and with the explanation that I was attempting to walk without the brace; the leg brace was soon removed. I remember when I started to take the leg brace off; my mother would get upset. In our home, we had a long wooden coffee table that was at my level as far as standing. I would use this table as my support and limp around this table as music played on my father's stereo. My family told me later I would do this for hours it seemed; just 'dance' around this table. I do remember this activity. It made me happy with the music an all. What possessed me to do this, I do not know. Looking back on it all, I think I saw everyone else walking around me, so why shouldn't I walk.

My parents continued to bask in my progress and growth and put my surgeries and near brush with death behind them. The years that followed were very normal for me. My parents began to get back to family life, which consisted of focusing on raising their four boys. Other than the occasional doctors appointment, which became less frequent during this time, I was growing up and progressing as a young boy. By age 5, I was wearing my scoliosis brace for most of the day, while doing normal boyhood activities. I had by this time adapted a sort of limp-like walk. With my left leg a little shorter than my right, a limp was apparent. I enjoyed playing around in the yard with our many different pets. I helped my father who would work on home improvement projects. I would swim and fish in the lake behind our home with my brothers and neighborhood kids. Even though I had a noticeable limp when I walked, my parents remember me getting around and being pretty mobile. Looking back at all the family photos of this time in my history, I was genuinely a happy child. I would have to return to the doctor every few months in order to adjust my brace and have a round of x-rays to access the scoliosis.

In 1974, my family moved from Dunwoody, Georgia to Roswell Georgia. We moved to a larger home more ac-commodating to my family. It was around this time that I really remember public school and all that it entailed. So here I go, at the age of 6, off to the bus stop at the end of our street. I waited each morning with my brother Kevin for the big yellow bus to take us to school. Looking back at this time, it was very difficult for me to deal with riding on the bus and going to school. I imagined I looked very strange with this scoliosis brace on; and the other kids on the bus and in my grade responded to it. Everyone wanted to know what this brace was and why I wore it. Some of them made fun of it, some just avoided me. It was a painful experience for a 5-year-old to endure. I despised going to school during these years. I basically was labeled handicapped. It was very hard to adjust socially. I wore turtleneck sweaters and heavy jackets just to disguise my situation. Children can be very cruel with situations that they do not understand. I endured this constant wrath of judgment. During recess, I was only able to stand around and observe. The doctors had given my parents instructions for no body contact sports at all, as this could jeopardize my delicate condition.

We moved again in 1976, to Beaumont, Texas as my father took another job in a different industry. This move was challenging for me as it meant staring over in a new environment. I would have to readjust with new friends and a new school. Just when I had fit in with the public school society, I had to change locations and start all over again. With dislike of the first days of school, I would plead with my mother to let me go to school initially without my brace. I wanted to at least go to school with a normal looking appearance. I remember those as good days when I went without my brace. My fellow classmates treated me as normal.

With moving to a new part of the country, comes a new set of doctors for me to deal with. I really don't remember the doctors and specialist in Houston, Texas. We had to travel there from Beaumont to the numerous medical centers of Houston, Texas. I do not really remember any specific doctor that was extraordinary during this time period. They all had muted faces and no outstanding or memorable personalities. If they had, I would have remembered them. All I remember were the white coats and the cold offices. No one ever spoke to me about my condition; they just addressed my parents. My physical conditions were basically guarded and monitored during these years. I just remember growing up during these following two years in a fantastic environment. We had a rather large house in a subdivision just outside of Beaumont, Texas. This was our first house with a swimming pool; in which I put to constant use. This year and half to two year period that we as a family live in Beaumont ended up being a comfortable time for me. School once again, had it challenges with wearing a brace. Most of the fellow students and teachers were very understanding. I had a couple close friends I confided in and spent most of my time with them. I did as much of the normal boyhood activities that I could. I rode bikes, took care of our many pets, and swam in the pool, and got into fishing the waterways that ran through our subdivision.

I just vaguely remember going to the doctor during this time. Having to take a day and drive to Houston, Texas was inconvenient enough for me. Missing a day of school for me was met with many questions upon my return. I felt some of my friends has a genuine concern for me. I shared with them my situation. This was good to tell them what was going on with me; it would allow a sort of protectionism to prevail. Whenever I was made fun of, a close friend of mine would always be in earshot; and come immediately to my aid.

I remember on one occasion, a fellow classmate by the name of Chris would on many occasions make fun of me either for how I walked or how ridiculous he thought I looked in my brace. One of my friends would always intervene to stop the bullying. I recall Chris was a rather big kid for his age with the bully-like personality to go with it. Needless to say, I was not his only prey among my classmates. He had been in trouble on several occasions with other students. Through out the school year I had several interactions with him in which my teacher was made aware of the problem. Nothing was really ever done to him other than a verbal reprimand. I told my father about this kid always making fun of me. My father, being the honest man that he is, told me that I should always defend myself when threatened. Make it a point to not start any trouble, but if trouble comes at you, defend your honor.

On one day when I was about 8 years old, I was put to the test. Chris was out at the monkey bars on the school grounds. I had to pass by him to go to the back of the field. I do not remember what he said to me when I walked by him as he was hanging from the bars. I told him to stop teasing me; he had already been in trouble in the past for teasing me. He told me to come over to him and make him stop. I told him that I would not fight him, as I am unable to with a brace on. And then I thought to myself, 'What's

WHERE DOES THE FIGHT COME FROM?

he going to do me? I have a brace on. 'Metal bars surround me in this brace'. As I got closer to him, he pushed me away from him and then called me "crippled". He then jumped up in front of me and reached for the bars to hang. He then continued his verbal bashing as he was hanging there in front of me.

I do not know what came over me, I just thought of my honor and what my father said to me. I then just launched back with my good leg and kicked him between his legs. He fell to the ground like stone on a pond. He laid on the ground with his face all red, moaning in agony. I just walked away back to the classroom.

Getting back to the classroom, I told the teacher what happened; within the hour, I was at the principal's office having to explain myself. My parents were notified, and they had to come down to the school. Long story short, I was just reprimanded by the school. My father later told me he was proud of me. Chris and I later apologized to each other and became decent friends after that incident.

At the end of 1977, my father came home one day and informed me that we were going to move to New Jersey so that he could take on a new job with a different company. A few months later we moved. I had to say goodbye to many of my friends who I had grown accustom to. Here I was again in the same predicament; had to start over in a new place, new school, and new social setting.

28

CHAPTER 4:
FITTING IN THE CROWD

Before I could blink an eye it seemed, I was in a new town. We had relocated to northern New Jersey, to a small historic town called Chester. This was a place in the countryside of New Jersey where farms and horse stables dotted long country roads. Many of the homes in that area were historic. Chester was a made of a main street through a town from circa late 1800's; it looked like an old movie set to me. All the old white churches and on cemeteries at the edge of town made you realize when passing through that there exists some valuable history in this town.

The year was 1978 and I had experienced so much in my first decade of life. I had a few months to get use to my new surroundings before I started back to school. My brothers Kevin and Tim moved with us as my oldest brother, Mike stayed in Beaumont, Texas to work.

This move to New Jersey marked a time for big changes for me. It was a time when I started to grow physically and mentally. A move to a new state also meant a new battalion of doctors in New York City. My scoliosis began to progress in a negative way. I was referred to a few doctors at Sloan-Kettering Cancer Center and New York Hospital. My pediatric cancer specialist was Dr. Lawrence

Helson, and my doctor who was in charge of monitoring my scoliosis was Dr. David Levine from New York Hospital for Special Surgery. In doing my research for this book I found out that these two doctors still practice to this day.

After my initial evaluations by these specialists, I was then placed on a regular check-up schedule. The check up included blood work, scoliosis exam, and a barrage of x-rays. This type of appointment took most of a day in New York to accomplish.

A profound change happened to me at the age of 10. One day, my father and uncle took me with them to The Olympic Racquetball and Health Club, in Randolph, New Jersey. At this stage in my development, I was required to wear the Scoliosis brace 20 to 23 hours a day. Up until that time, I had never heard of racquetball; I figured it was something like tennis but inside a room. When I saw racquetball played for the first time, I was immediately attracted to the game. I walked around the club and watched each court with great enthusiasm to try this sport. Having not been allowed to participate in any sports, I was very anxious to do some form of physical activity. The doctors in charge of my care at the time frowned on the idea of any type of body contact sport, as it would possibly jeopardize my health. Needless to say, I was attracted to racquetball. So while my father and uncle were playing, I went to the front desk and asked if I could borrow a racquet and a ball to hit by myself in an unlit court next to my father and uncle. I don't recall asking my father if I could go out and hit by myself; I just went out there with my brace on and tried to hit the ball around. What I like about racquetball was the court was like a box. If you hit a ball while inside a racquetball court, the ball has a tendency to come back at you. It was basically an activity that I could do by myself that was some form of exercise. I ended that day hitting the ball around with my father and having him explain to me how the game is played. This was how my racquetball experience began.

From that point on, I would go with my father to the health club and while he lifted weights, I would find an open court and hit the ball around. I would observe others playing and watch the different skill levels in action. I started to take my brace off to play, as the structure and function of the brace were not conducive to physical activity. Looking back on that time, wearing a scoliosis brace while having your body try to grow at the same time was painful. As I stated before, it was like wearing a medieval torture device. The structure of a scoliosis brace was to support and inhibit movement of the spine. I remember the pads of the brace, which were located in the pelvic, and lumbar areas would rub and dig into my skin. I had to wear a thin t-shirt under the brace to protect my skin. This brace had to be adjusted and refitted about every 4 months during my growing years. So this brace, in my opinion, had to be taken off if I was going to play racquetball.

It was around 1980, and racquetball was becoming a very popular sport. I was really getting into it. I went with my father to the health club about 3 to 5 times a week to play. I just generally felt better after playing. My spine was at such a curvature, that pain was just a part of my day. Racquetball changed that for me. I remember going to New York, Sloan Kettering Cancer Center to meet one of my many specialists, Dr. David Levine. He was in charge of monitoring my progress during this time of my life. I told him I have been taking the brace off and playing racquetball. He stated to just be careful, and that he was proud of my notable improvements.

Scoliosis is measured in degrees of severity of the curvature of the spine. In a perfect world there should be a 0 degree curvature in the horizontal plain of positioning. By June 3rd, 1980, my lumbar scoliosis curve was holding at 25+ degrees. The doctors recommended that I be fitted with a new polyethylene scoliosis brace, which fit more like a corset made of plastic. It could be worn under the clothing and had no metal bars or chin apparatus. I liked the idea because no one would know if I was wearing a brace. My condition however, was sending me down the path to surgery if I got any worse.

CHAPTER 4: Fitting in the Crowd

In June 1980, during one of my doctor exams, it was determined that my scoliosis was progressing over 25 degrees. Dr. David Levine suggested that I return in 6 months and be re-examined and fitted for a new type of polythetylene (plastic) underarm brace that would replace the Milwaukee brace I was wearing. I like this idea because it was a new style of brace that you wear under clothing, with no metal bars and such. It was upon my return for a check up in December 1980, I found out that after an examination that I had extremely high blood pressure. The doctors thought that due to the lumbar scoliosis, the shape of my rib cage might change and impede organ function. It was discovered at this time, that one of my kidneys near the tumor site might not be functioning properly. This possible lack of function was the cause of my increase in blood pressure. During this period, I felt fine; I did not understand why the doctors were making a huge issue of it. They informed my parents and I that I would be admitted to New York Hospital in January 1981 for 3 to 4 week stay in order to evaluate the high blood pressure and hypertension. I was devastated; I fought with my parents to not take me there. Needless to say, I wanted Christmas and the holiday season to last for longer than it did that year.

Returning back to school at the beginning of the New Year was difficult. I had to go into school and inform my teachers that I would be gone for a few weeks. I collected all my homework and told a few friends that I was heading to the hospital in New York for tests and observation. Little did I know that this experience in the hospital would have such an influence on my life. I was excited that I was getting a new type of brace. I was however disappointed that I would be hospitalized for so long, when I felt great. On the 6th of January 1981, I was admitted on a cold an icy winter day to New York Hospital. My parents reassured me that they would come see as much as possible as we lived over an hour away.

I was given a room on the fourth floor in the pediatric section of the hospital. The room was a rather large by today's standards. It had two windows with a small bench in between. It was a bright room since the sun was beaming in, with the morning New York skyline as a background. With light colored walls and two beds with a curtain between, the room seamed pleasant. I chose the bed furthest from the entrance of the room, near the windows. It was upon walking into this room that a unique smell came to my senses. It was a mixture of cleaning solutions and sweat with a faint smell of bad cafeteria food. It was as if the person who stayed in this room had something bad happen to them, only then it was disguised with bleach and ammonia to not reveal what took place. I was unaware at the time that people take their last breaths in these rooms. Their last moments on this earth are spent here surrounded by their loved ones. These rooms are where the final battles are fought. I settled in my room in a calm manor as to not disturb anything, as my parents helped me unpack. They each took turns going to talk with the nurses and sign paperwork. They kept reassuring me that I would be fine. We said our good byes and my parents traveled home back to the countryside with the promise to call me later and check on me.

As I got settled in, a realization came to me that I am 12 years old and alone in this huge hospital surrounded by strangers, in a room with a strange smell, and not knowing what tomorrow will bring. With many questions swimming around in mind, my body began to ache. I went and sat on the sterile white sheets of my bed and looked out the window. Within a few hours of occupying this room, I was greeted with a new roommate; he took up residence, occupying the other half of the room.

After a few hours of watching the TV in my room, a nurse by the name of Jean came in and informed me of the protocol for my stay. She took me on a tour of the 4th floor. It really began to sink in with me as she told me about what goes on here. As she told me about the details of my daily schedule, we walked down the halls. We passed by many hospital personnel and other patients on the ward. I remember seeing many of the young patients in gowns shuffling up and down the halls with IV's in their arms. Some were just laying on gurneys with family members around them. They were all in huddles like a quarterback giving his teammates the instructions for the big play to win the game. No one made eye contact with me as Jean and I continued the tour of this place where battles are won and lost. She told me that all of the children in this section of the hospital were fighting cancer in some form or another. They had surgery and were recovering, or were under treatment and awaiting surgery. The nurse informed me that most of the children here are extremely sick. As my tour continued, she showed me where I was going to eat. Jean took me to a small florescent-lit room with yellow walls with a few tables.

An old television played cartoons in one corner of the room as three or four children sat like skeletons with an IV in their arms, dressed in hospital gowns. They ate from their trays with weak arms and not making eye contact as my tour continued.

During the day in this place, I always heard crying off in the distance. Crying was mixed in with announcements over the intercom of someone paging a doctor or staff member. As I discussed before, this place had a smell to it that is difficult to describe. Along with the odors of cleaning solutions, old cafeteria food, and poor ventilation, the whole floor had an additional smell like something was in a state of decay. All hospitals in general just have a distinct smell to them. To this day, if I even walk into a hospital, I feel uneasy. Even If I am there for the birth of a child or to see a friend, I feel strange.

The nurse continued to inform me that I would have to get up at 6AM everyday and go to an exam room everyday and be weighed, examined, and collect a urine sample from me. So here I am, thrown into the middle of all this. When the tour ended, I went back to my room and called my father. I told him I wanted out of here as soon as possible. I was *not* sick. He reassured me and to me to sit tight and follow the staffs directions.

It was torture trying to sleep in a place where all this is going on around you. It only got really quiet after midnight. I remember laying in bed looking out my window out into the city wondering about myself and could I handle my stay at this hospital. I wondered about the people in the buildings across from me, what where they going through? New York Hospital was a huge place surrounded by smaller buildings. Directly across from my building was a mental hospital with a courtyard separating us. I would think to myself, 'How bad does it have to get to be admitted to that place?' I then eased off to sleep only to get a few quiet hours of calm.

The next morning at 6AM, I woke up for the morning routine of blood work, urine collection and a physical exam. I remember a doctor and a couple staff members accomplish this task as a joint effort as a number of patients proceeded through a doorway; I was dressed in just a hospital gown and underwear. You get processed through the line like a cow in a slaughterhouse. No one person really talked to me as I waited to get processed; they just took collections and measurements. They would just nod and mumble it seems as they wrote their discoveries on a clipboard; and give directions to move on. They kept the room so uncomfortably cold. Upon my arrival at the hospital, my blood pressure was taken 10 or so times a day. My high blood pressure readings started to go down after a few days of being hospitalized. Why? It was never discovered why that happened.

My first two weeks in the hospital consisted of a variety of tests. They would perform tests and scans on me and take more x-rays. On one occasion, I was not given any food for about 6 hours, then had to swallow a charcoal tasting black dye and then transported to a lab and x-rayed every two minutes to determine kidney function. The dye made me sick; I spent the rest of the evening throwing up. I just felt like a guinea pig in a lab. I began to trust no one on the staff. This was my regiment and it was horrible. I remember I could not brush my teeth enough to get that charcoal taste out of my mouth.

CHAPTER 4: FITTING IN THE CROWD

As soon as I returned to my room from these various tests, I would change out of the hospital gown and shower. I would then put my street cloths back on; within my mind, if I had my regular cloths on, I was *not sick*. I protested wearing pajamas and a robe all day. Having my street cloths just made me feel better. I would look for nurse Jean as I confided in her. She would just make everything bearable for me. She took the time to listen to me. I would also reach out to my family. When I had bad experiences at the hospital, I would call my mother and father out of despair to find some comfort in their words.

My family would come see me as much as they could during the week and on the weekends. My mother brought many cards and well wishes from my friends and other family members, which was a nice reprieve from all that was happening to me. My fellow classmates all signed a big card for me wishing me well! I enjoyed that. At some point during my stay, I had to start on all the schoolwork that was assigned to me. On a day when I had no tests, nurse Jean took me upstairs to a library/play area for smaller children on the 9th floor to get started on my schoolwork.

On one of my visits up there I met a 6-year-old girl who was coloring at one of the tables. I talked to her and her mother for a while. Her mother told me she had leukemia, and was in the battle of her life. This little girl had no hair, very thin, but still an amazing smile on her face. She sat and colored and would draw a variety of pictures. I talked with her and helped her color a few pictures. She told me about her cancer with her descriptions only a child can explain. We laughed and colored as we passed the time. I saw her there on numerous occasions, and then at one point, she was gone. After not seeing her or her mother, I asked the attendant working in the activities room if she had gone home. With quiet words, the woman informed me that the little girl had passed away a few days ago.

This news disturbed me greatly. This was my first experience with death in this hospital. It was at this point I realized that some people did not make it through their stay at this place. In the following two weeks, several other young people died while being treating for their various conditions. My roommate even died during the night after he went upstairs for a brain tumor operation. He came back down from surgery to our room, I was awoken during the night when the alarms went off from his side of the curtain divided room. The nurses took me out of the room to an adjacent room. I watch from the doorway of my new room as numerous staff and doctors rushed to his aid. Within the hour, he was deceased. Taking all this in was very difficult for me. It made sleeping a challenge through my additional nights. What would happen to my family if I died here? What if I died here with no one around me but "white coats." I started to worry about my kidneys, my scoliosis and cancer. My parents would be devastated to loose me in a place like this.

The next morning, with my early morning routine complete, I ventured down to my old room to get the rest of my belongings. As I walked in the room, my room-mate's section of the room had all been cleaned and arranged. Once again, the room was freshly cleaned, so the smell of bleach and ammonia was in the air, ready for the next patient. There was no trace of my roommate, as all his personal affects were gone. Death had occurred in that room, so I avoided it the rest of my stay. I called my parents on many occasions and pleaded to come get me out of this place where people die. I went through another few days of test and x-rays. I was also fitted with the new brace for my scoliosis. It was a plastic-like corset brace hidden under my cloths. The best thing was that no one knew I had it on.

I have to mention the food that I was provided while hospitalized at New York Hospital was absolutely nasty. My diet was strictly controlled for salt intake since I was incurring kidney and blood pressure problem. I was feed a no-salt diet with limited food choices, and expected to flourish. I actually lost a large amount of weight and also became sick with a flu-like illness my last 10 days of hospitalization. I hated the food that consisted of macaroni and cheese, grilled cheese sandwiches, and some kind of meat called beef with no sauces. It was disgusting. I could not wait to get out and have a big hamburger and fries. Needless to say I did not fare well on their food regiment. When I found out that I was getting released from the hospital within 48 hours, I was overcome with joy. My thoughts and experiences there in that hospital definitely changed me. I grew up on many levels; mentally, physically, and not to mention spiritually. When my father came down the hall to the nurses' station where I was waiting, a feeling of excitement and freedom rushed through me….I had made it, my stay was over.

I said goodbye to the many doctors and nurses that treated me with compassion. They all signed a book for me filled with well wishes. Upon release from the hospital, my father took me to the Empire Diner in The Village to eat. He told me to order whatever I wanted. I ordered a hamburger and fries with a large sweet tea; and it never tasted so good. He told me he was proud of me for enduring that experience, as we toasted our sweet teas. It was one of my great father-son moments.

It was never explained why my blood pressure returned to normal only a few weeks after being hospitalized. I went through all the tests and exams and nothing came of it. I was just glad to be out of that place. I looked at the stay as a positive experience because I was fitted with a new brace. I liked this brace because I was told to wear it for fewer hours a day and it was hidden under my cloths. Looking back on that time in the hospital, I realized that I grew up a little on the maturity level. I saw many things that the public never sees. It was like I grew up mentally in 4 weeks. My other focus was to get back on the racquetball court as soon as possible. My father promised me we would play later in the week.....*and we did!*

Getting back on a racquetball schedule was important for me. All of the members greeted me back to the racquetball club with open arms as they found out I had been hospitalized. It meant so much to me that I was missed on the racquetball courts. I had created a bond from that point on with many of the club members. Many weeks had to pass before I was back up to speed as far as racquetball. I had lost a good bit of weight and stamina being hospitalized. My mother made sure I ate extra helpings in the following weeks to put on weight. The fact that I was basically in the hospital for almost a month gave me a better appreciation for the sun. It felt great getting back to doing yard work and experiencing the outdoors. Even if the day was cold, it felt great to have the sunshine down on me. Upon returning home from the hospital, I made it a point to be outside in nature as much as could. It continues for me as an adult, to enjoy all that nature has to offer. It seems that even when I have difficult days, how a walk in the woods, a walk around the lake, or a stroll on the beach alone, tends to make everything calm.

Character cannot be developed in ease and quiet. Only through experience of trial and suffering can the soul be strengthened, ambition inspired, and success achieved."
~Helen Keller

CHAPTER 5:
MATURITY

I do not really remember a finite time when I thought of myself as an adult. The hospital stay that I endured as a 12 year-old boy was a pinnacle moment that is engrained in my mind. That experience alone brought a sense of maturity to me. I had to handle a lot of issues at such a fast pace; it made me realize I was heading on to adulthood. There is that time in one's history where one legally becomes an adult at age 18 or legal to consume alcohol at age 21. Reaching those ages was not a big deal to me in my mind. I felt that I had already become an adult much earlier than my age indicated. For a male, physically at age 18, you are a man. I do not really remember my transition to manhood; it just happened one day. There was a time when I thought I was a boy; I did not have much to worry about. I played in the woods, built tree forts on our property, and rode bikes, and collected insects and stamps. But while this was going on, I was always thinking about my health and wellness. As far back as I can remember.... I was always thinking about the dynamics of my medical condition.

Throughout my life, cancer and the medical appointments were the mainstay. When I was exposed to death and dying during my stay at New York Hospital, made me realize that I was unique. This exposure to cancer and all that it entails made me realized that I had a tremendous task of addressing cancer and dealing with the after affects, and processing all that I had experienced.

Cancer to me seemed like a "black cloud" that hung over me through my formative years. I tried my best to ignore it; but it always seemed to visit me in my dreams at night. I would sometimes dream about my situation and think what would I do if cancer were 'asleep' inside of me, hiding like a thief in the night. At some point…maybe my next doctor visit, it would awaken and show up on some exam or test. What would I do?? How would I react? How many more surgeries would I need to deal with it? How long would it take to kill me?

I kept these thoughts swimming around in my mind; I just did not discuss them with anyone, not even my family. Many of my friends would ask me about my noticeable limp or antalgic lean when I walked. I only discussed my condition with a few close friends. I had a feeling of embarrassment about physical appearance. When some-one would ask me about why I walked 'funny', I would make up a story like I fell an injured my ankle or leg; and he or she would cease thier inquiry. I tried my best to appear normal. I had been through so much scrutiny as a youngster going through the public school system. It is tough to express the loneliness one feels when you are the point of a joke. Children can be overwhelming with their cruelty. By just wearing a Scoliosis brace of any kind, I took on the label of pariah; and was looked upon as handicapped. At some point in my life that brace which was shackled to my identity and me…. had to come off.

I continued to wear my new brace less and less the following year. I increased the frequency of racquetball. My over-all health began to improve. It was around the age of 13 that I mentally thought I had conquered my condition. All I had to do was to continue to improve and I would stay out of the hands of the surgeon. The relocation from Beaumont, Texas to Chester, New Jersey, allowed us easy access to the many of the top doctors in the fields relating to my condition. I had to venture to New York every few months to see this or that specialist. I despised going to see these people in white coats. It was as if these appointments to see these people interrupted my own recovery in my mind. My goal was to not have the need to see these 'white coats'; I thought if I stayed away from them, I was getting better.

Looking back in New Jersey worked out very well for me. My parents bought about 5 acres of land out in the woods in the northern section of the state. My father had a corporate job at an office in Newark, New Jersey. He commuted the one-hour car ride to from our home to work each day. I enjoyed living out in the woods on our property. We had a sizable home, decent acreage; and our property bordered state owned property, which consisted of hundreds of acres. There were streams, trails, wildlife and lakes to fish. A few residents in the area had horses and stables. I enjoyed the solitude. I had a few close friends who lived near by; they were just a bike ride away. Each day I would come home from school, do the miscellaneous chores that my parents asked of me, and then I would venture out and explore. My friends and I would ride bikes all through the woods, go fishing, and we even built a tree fort. In the evenings I would join my father at the racquetball club and play. It was just a memorable, simple time in my life.

Every few months, like an ominous date with destiny, my mother would inform me of my upcoming doctor appointment. I would always argue…"Why? I feel fine". I would have to go to school and get my assignments for the following day that I would miss. School was the last thing on my mind with an upcoming doctor appointment on my horizon. At this age of 13, I also realized that I was in a guarded situation with regards to my physical condition. I had read about cancer, I had read about scoliosis; I knew that there was a chance cancer could come back later on in life, and that surgery for scoliosis may be inevitable.

WHERE DOES THE FIGHT COME FROM?

For me, going to a simple doctor appointment at one of the top hospitals in the United States was very intimidating not to mention over whelming. Sitting in each of the waiting rooms and seeing all of the conditions and afflictions of the variety of patients made me more aware of my own battle. I would silently repeat to myself that ' I am not sick, I am not sick. I should not even be here'. These patients were worse off than me. This was the psychology I used on myself.

Why? ....I don't know.

To miss school was a big deal to me. As I stated before, to miss school raised questions among my classmates. One of my close friends at the time was Randy. He was one of the few people I confided in, as he was a very grounded individual. He was a very generous and understanding person. He came from a wealthy family and lived about 4 miles from me. Looking back, he was not judgmental or disconcerting in any way. I remember he would tell me just to go the appointments and *get them done; I would be fine.* — He was just a good friend to have during that time in my life.

Each summer, Randy's family would retire to their beach residence at the New Jersey shore and stay down there for most of the summer. He invited me down on several occasions, but my schedule would not allow. By the time I was 14 and heading into my high school years, I had been invited down to the beach multiple times, but my mother had me decline for one reason or another. Later on, a final invite and my subsequent decline of that offer would affect me in the following weeks and years to come.

CHAPTER 6:
My Own Mortality

By 1982, with the infamous hospital stay behind me, my doctor appointments becoming less frequent, I felt I was well on track to my own recovery. My years in the 7th and 8th grades went by uneventful. I concentrated on playing as much racquetball as possible as my skill level was improving. My body physically began to grow. I was wearing my brace mainly at night, or when I was experiencing back pain. Having a curved spine while at the same time your body is trying to grow, means that for most of the day, back pain became part of the equation.

The only time this would subside was when I was on the racquetball court moving around. I soon began to participate in local tournaments as my skill improved. As long as I was clothed, I looked completely normal, besides the visible limp when I walked. On the racquetball court I moved around with decent agility. My whole goal was to appear as normal looking as possible. People would come up to me at the racquetball club and tournaments and ask me about my limp. I would still resort back to my story of a 'twisted ankle'. I said anything to get the focus off of me. I was still so uncomfortable discussing anything about my condition. The only way I could 'hide' from everything was to be on the racquetball court. Something inside of me felt relieved when I was on the court. I could escape from reality for a time just by being on the court itself. At this point in my life, my desire to become a top racquetball player was driven by my ambition.

I was playing local tournaments in both my age division and my skill division. In the beginning, I lost many of these events in the first rounds of play. This was a big character builder for me. I got discouraged from time to time, but as time passed, I somehow began to gain momentum and progress with an occasional positive result. I would last a few rounds of play and take third or fourth. This little bit of positive progression on the racquetball court gave me the drive to want to become a really good player and defy the odds.

My parents were the consummate supporters for me with my racquetball. My father allowed me to get better equipment as my skill and interest improved. Another aspect of becoming a skilled player in racquetball comes respect. I think on some level, respect and admiration was one of my goals. I wanted to be known as a great player.

During this developmental time in my life I began to grow socially in school. I had developed a few great friendships that I would later look back on with a genuine feeling. Middle school crushes and eighth grade dances became the new focus of my attention instead of my studies. I really did not think of cancer, my doctor appointments, or my scoliosis; I found it easy to just wall it off in my mind. I did this because I saw myself as a normal kid in middle school getting ready for high school and all that it entailed. It felt like I had my own identity because I was now semi popular in school, and decent at racquetball; I recall feeling free from the grip of my condition.

By the end of summer of 1982, I was heading into high school. I was looking forward to it, as I had to go to a larger school in the neighboring town of Mendham, New Jersey. My freshman year of high school went by very fast for me. I socially stayed with a couple close friends to handle the overwhelming change in school environments. My friend Randy and a few others tried to get as many classes together as possible. The school was rather large with students shipped in from surrounding towns. So it was safe to say that there was a feeling of social safety staying close to your friends. I had no problems my freshman year of school. I did not wear my brace to school; I only wore it at night and on the weekends. Due to my fragile spine, I was exempted from most of gym class. I would go to the library and read. I would find confidence and peace in working in the yard with my father on the weekends, cutting grass, planting in our garden, and doing chores. It was after these tasks that my back would hurt, and I would voluntarily wear my brace for support, but only around the house.

On one of my last visits to my doctors that summer, I remember my orthopedic doctor informing my parents and I that due to the condition of my scoliosis and the possible progression of the curve as I matured; they recommended Herrington Rod Surgery for my lower spine. This is a surgical procedure in which two metal rods on either side of a patient's spine. The rods are then wired to each vertebrae involved in the curvature. For me, the procedure would add to the support of my spine for the rest of my life. I did some research at the time while doing book reports for school about this type of surgery. It sounded painful to me as well as looked so invasive. If I had it done, I would have less range of motion in my spine and therefore would not be able to bend or twist normally. I would sit up *perfectly* straight. This would put me back into a situation of looking different, which I so despised.

So now I had to face that I may go back to meet the hands of surgeon; I was not yet out of the harms way. My parents told me to just forget about it and focus on what was important to me now.

It was a wait and see situation. So my situation was guarded. I returned to school following that doctor appointment telling my friends that all was well. I decided to forget about what the doctors told me. I just went back to playing racquetball and focused on friends and school.

It was now the summer of 1983. With my freshman year of high school behind me, I mainly played racquetball and enjoyed being off from school. It was at this time that my parents informed me that we will be moving to Dallas, Texas so that my father could start on a new business venture. In fact he said that he was going to be making frequent trips to Texas to look for a new home and begin working. He would be absent most of that summer. My brothers all lived in Atlanta, Georgia by this time. It was just my mother and I who stayed in New Jersey until my father set us up in Texas. I was now faced with the last summer I would have in New Jersey. I focused on being with friends and playing as much racquetball as time allowed. I was now the man of the house while my father was away.

Yard maintenance and upkeep were now my solo re-sponsibility. My mother was working for a chiropractor in town in order to make ends meet. This was the first time in my life that I was exposed to chiropractic as a therapy option for my scoliosis. I received treatments from Dr. Alan Marr for a short period of time before we eventually moved away. At the time, I was so jaded by the sight of a doctor, any doctor, that I did not have an appreciation of chiropractic until later on in my life.

CHAPTER 6: My Own Mortality

I spent most of the summer working around the house, cutting the grass, taking care of the pets, and cutting the neighbors lawn. Randy had again invited me down to their family beach house early in the month of August for a week stay. I asked my mother if I could go once again for a last visit with my friend and his family at the New Jersey shore. I told Randy that I would be moving to Texas in the next few months, so now would be the best time to come down to the shore as it would be my last summer in New Jersey.

The problem came when my mother denied me permission to go to the New Jersey shore once again. I was so upset that I called my father in Texas; I begged him to override my mother's decision. He told me after much discussion that he had to stand behind my mother's choice to not let me go; after all my mother was in charge of me, my father was a thousand miles away. I rode my bike over to Randy's house to hang out and shoot basketball. I told him my mother would not let me go. My mother never really told me why; looking back on it, I would call it a mother's intuition. Randy and I rode bikes and shot basketball in the driveway to make the best of our eventual final day. We talked about school life for the upcoming sophomore year, girls, and how we would stay in touch after I moved. As I left his house, I remember it was a Thursday, we agreed that we would see each other at the beginning of September, when school would resume. We said goodbye to each other and I told him to enjoy the beach.

I remember riding my bike home feeling really mad that I would have to miss this opportunity to go to the beach as these were the last remaining months in New Jersey for me. I basically moped around the house that weekend, as I continued to dwell on my mother's decision. On Sunday morning, Kurt who was Randy's cousin called me and told me he had something very bad to tell me. Audibly upset, Kurt told me on Saturday, Randy, his brother Rick, sister Jill, father Joe, and a family friend, and two pilots had all crashed into the ocean on a site seeing tour of the coast in a tour helicopter. Kurt told me to turn on the TV and check the news. I could not believe what I was hearing. I turned on the 5 o'clock news and sure enough; there it was. It was unclear in the report who was dead and who was alive. It turns out that Randy, his father, and a family friend, as well as two pilots had died in the crash. Rick and Jill, his brother and sister were in intensive care fighting for their lives. I was devastated. I went upstairs to tell me mother of this accident that took so many lives.

My mother just embraced me and we cried.....it was one of the toughest moments for me to handle. In discussing the situation with my mother, we both soon realized that I too would have been on that helicopter. I could have shared the same fate. My mother wept even more; we were just numb from hearing all this. I could not believe my friend was gone. I just saw him a few days prior, we shot basketball together; this nightmare could not be true.

It was like time stopped for me. I had that Monday to think about what just happened. I thought about my own mortality; I could have been on that helicopter with them. My parents would have been devastated if they lost me in this way. My mother was right in her decision to not let me go.

The following Tuesday I was going to a wake in a funeral home for Randy and his family. I told my mother I wanted to go to pay my respects. I remember the ride over to the wake was quiet and calm.

As I looked out the side window, glancing up into the trees, which lined our route to the funeral home, I went through all my memories of Randy. I lost a good friend; and I would never see him again. My thoughts of Randy's mother and older bother were filled with questions. How are they going to handle this loss? With tears streaming down my face, I just stared up into the trees as they passed, seeing the occasional bird fly out as our car whisked passed.

My mother explained to me what to expect at a wake, as we did not know if the casket would be open or closed.

WHERE DOES THE FIGHT COME FROM?

When I walked in to the viewing room at the funeral home; I just remember everything going quiet for me. The room was adorned with flowers, soft music, and low light as I walked up to the open casket; and there was my friend. I just did not want to believe he was gone from this earth until I saw him. To my recollection, Randy was dressed in a suit; his hands were crossed over his body with rosary beads draped on top of them. He did not look real to me. He had died of massive internal injuries and was basically intact. His face looked like a plastic mannequin as he lay there. I went to view his father's body briefly, and then went to give my condolences to Randy's mother.

She made the choice to stay back at the beach condo and did not go on the helicopter tour. I went back to see Randy one final time. I told him "goodbye" as my eyes welled up. I touched him on the hand, paused for a moment, and turned and walked out of the room to meet my waiting mother.

My mother's eyes were welled up from crying, as I too felt tense from all that was upon me. We left the funeral home for the long ride back to our house. I apologized to her for getting upset for them not allowing me to go down to the beach, I just felt horrible. The loss of Randy took something from me; it took my innocence. An understanding fell upon me that life is so fragile. I did not want to believe my friend was gone even though I just saw his body. The following day was the funeral that I chose to not attend, I felt it would be too much for me to handle. To my recollection, I stayed home that entire day. Later on in the week, we were informed that Jill, Randy's older sister finally passed away from here injuries. This news just added to my further depressive state.

Surviving many surgeries, fighting cancer, and then the decision to not go to the beach and become involved in a helicopter accident. I thought of myself as I was saved from these demises for a reason. Questions began for me about my own mortality and purpose in life. These are difficult topics for a 14 year-old to mentally process.

To this day, I never forget my friend Randy and his family. I remember him mostly in the month of August. He died on August 14th, 1983. August is the month of my birthday as well as the loss of a good friend. It is also the month that I celebrate a time of maturity that was both very difficult and empowering for me as young man. My life changed in that month of my 14th year on this earth. I keep Randy in a place in my mind that I can easily access; I never forget him. I made a point to live a prosperous life *for him*; for his was taken too soon.

I headed back to school for my sophomore year that September 1984. My parents informed that we would be moving to Dallas, Texas before Christmas. This meant more changes, a new environment, and a new school, were coming my way. I recall it was different going back to school and never seeing Randy walk those halls again. Many of my friends who new him discussed him less and less as the weeks passed. It was as if we were all looking for closure of some kind. I wrapped up my time in New Jersey saying goodbye to all my classmates before the school broke away for the holiday season. I exchanged addresses with many people in hopes of staying in contact with them. It was shortly after this, with our cars packed up, I was on my way to a new chapter in my life starting with a trip down the long road to Texas.

CHAPTER 7:
A New Beginning in Texas

We moved to an apartment in Arlington, Texas upon arriving back to the South. My father had us move into it due to our new house would not be finished with construction for several months. We later moved into a glorious home my father had custom built in a rather affluent part of Dallas called North Arlington. I immediately began looking for a place to play racquetball and get started back on a routine. I found an apartment complex near ours that had a court that I capitalized on quickly.

With this move to Arlington, came a new set of challenges for me again; new school, new people, and a new environment. I don't recall any problems for me going to a new school. I was 15 years old by this time. Wearing my scoliosis brace was now just a nighttime requirement. Having to not wear this brace at school at all made the transition easy for me. At this point in my development, the brace was becoming a tight fit as I began to grow. My parents began to let me take control of my medical prognosis from this time on in my life moving forward. After we moved into our new home, I quickly joined one of the racquetball clubs in town. I came to the realization that the more I played the sport, the better my back felt; consequently, the less and less I wore my brace. I soon gave up wearing the brace all together.

I was well aware of the fact that the doctors in New York informed my parents that I would most likely require back surgery to further support my spine after I finished growing. If I did not get the Herrington Rods installed by the surgeon, my situation would worsen. Something inside of me, I call it my intuition, did not believe this prediction. I became adamantly against this surgical option, as it would further physically handicap me. I began to trust in myself with my decisions. My thoughts moving forward that year were that I was *not* going back under the knife for any reason. Focusing on school, racquetball, and friends became the norm for me. I went against the past various medical recommendations to limit my physical activity in order to "protect" my physical condition.

Being physical and active meant that I felt better. I even started a lawn mowing business in our neighborhood. A mindset came over me to ignore my scoliosis at this point; I figured I had made it this far in life; why worry about the 'black cloud'. During these two years we lived in Texas, I had a renewed experience with chiropractic treatment. My mother took a job not far from our home at a chiropractic clinic. At some point, my mother recommended me to come in and get evaluated and treated. Back pain and headaches began to be an issue with me as I started to physically grow. I knew very little about how chiropractic care can become instrumental in assisting the body to maintain a healthy condition.

At the age of 16, right after I received my new drivers license, I drove myself out to this clinic in Irving, Texas. Upon entering the clinic, I was greeted by Dr. John Daugherty, who I immediately found to be a caring and compassionate person. From my past experiences with all the different medical personnel I had met through my years, initial meetings were always uncomfortable.

Dr. John was in his late 20's at the time. His demeanor and genuine concern for my case made a lasting impression on me. I basically knew very little about the abilities of chiropractic care in regards to scoliosis. My mother had already filled him in about my case, which he reassured me that he would very much like to provide me care. The frequency of pain that I was experiencing made me decide to let go of my negative experiences with doctors, and allow Dr. John to treat me.

After taking my x-rays and doing an examination, Dr. John reiterated with me that he could help alleviate some of the pain of scoliosis. The condition of my spine at this time was basically guarded. My spinal column assumed the shape of an "s", with the lower back portion having the highest degree of curvature.

WHERE DOES THE FIGHT COME FROM?

I thought to myself, as long as I don't have to go to a hospital for treatment, there was no blood involved, and no braces, I was going to give chiropractic care a try. So over the next several months, I was treated at Dr. John's clinic two and three times a week. I received not only chiropractic care, but also muscle treatments, and traction to try to counteract the effects of scoliosis. I also kept playing racquetball as much as I could, competing more in local tournaments. It was after several months of treatment, upon a re-physical examination, did it all come together. My over all condition improved marked by a decrease in the severity of my scoliosis. I was hit with a growth spurt at this time, which added to positive outcome. With this chiropractic care came a measurable improvement; I felt that I had better agility and my pain discomfort decreased. The combination of all this added to a higher self esteem for me, which was like turning over a new chapter in my life.

It was during my senior year of high school that I decided that I wanted to become a Doctor of Chiropractic. My experience and subsequent improvement drew me right to the chiropractic profession as an occupation. Having the ability to help someone in need is a powerful thing to possess. With all that had had endured, the medical people I had met along the way, influenced me in regards to my choice to become some kind of doctor.

CHAPTER 7: A NEW BEGINNING IN TEXAS

After meeting Dr. Alan Marr and Dr. John Daugherty and becoming a patient, I felt that it was easy to make a choice of an educational path to take. I set out during the fall of 1987 to set up a path to reach my educational goals. Most of my friends had left town to head to big schools all over the country. Right after high school graduation I decided to take a year off and just work on neighborhood lawn business and save some money in the process. I remember many of my friends saying that if you don't go to college right out of high school; you will never go. So while they all went off to dormitories in far-off colleges, I stayed home.

It was not until the fall of the following year that I decided to enter community college. The year was 1987; I entered community college to begin my next journey. High school was very easy for me. Looking back on those years, I wished I had tried harder. I was basically a B/C student. All my fellow students were worried about GPA and class placement; I could have cared less. I just could not wait to get out of school each day to go and run my lawn business. I really had an entrepreneurial agenda on my mind. I just enjoyed working outside, making a few bucks, and staying in good physical condition. At one point, I even hired friends of mine that had gone off to the big college their first year and failed out; and returned home.

College to me was rather intimidating starting off the first day, big campus, large crowds, packed classrooms. The initial couple semesters proved very difficult for me. I remember at one point sitting in a Biology 101 class and having the professor pass out our mid-term exam results. I received a grade of "D". I thought to myself; how am I going to get a chiropractic degree with this kind of result? I did two semesters of minimal college performance before I decided to stop going and re-evaluate. Looking back on that time from my current perspective, I just was not ready to handle the college experience. With the passing of time, and further life experience, that would soon change.

With a few poor grades under my belt, and a decision to discontinue school, I decided to focus on racquetball and working. I recall that my parents were not happy with my choice. Shortly after this event that my father informed me that we may be moving to Atlanta, Georgia to start a new business venture. Within a few months, I was relocated to Atlanta….another chapter had ended, and a new one had begun.

CHAPTER 8:
ATLANTA, GEORGIA

The year was now 1988, having moved to Atlanta, Georgia. I was ready for a new start. I immediately started a lawn care business. My knowledge of it from Texas made this process easy. Within a very short period of time I had a good size enterprise going in the neighborhood. With the relocation, came the opportunity to join a new health club to restart my racquetball regiment.

I had reached the 20-year mark of my life. It was at this point in time that I made a conscious decision to consider myself undoubtedly cured from cancer. Therefore, I did not seek out any new doctors to monitor my condition. After discussions with my mother and father, I was going to stay with the current physical condition of my body and forgo any further corrective surgery for my scoliosis. All I really worried about was protecting my low back from any kind of injury. In retro-spec my decision to forgo surgery was one of the best choices I could have made. Having the degree of scoliosis that I developed meant each day consists of a certain degree of back pain and stiffness. I was just pleased to have the physical mobility to freely move about. For the next year, racquetball, family and friends were my focus. Racquetball tournaments both local and regional consumed my weekends.

As I turned 21 years old, the realization came upon me to get started back on my college education. In my many discussions with my father, a higher education was always stressed as key to ones development. With my first attempt at college left my ego battered and bruised. It took another event to spark my interest and recalibrate my goals on obtaining a college degree.

Near the end of the summer of 1989, I was involved in a car accident. It was nothing major or life threatening; but the accident was enough to awaken a sleeping giant inside of me. That sleeping giant was the initiation of a different level of pain in my body. To put it in perspective, the human spinal column is equivalent to tall stack of teacups and saucers. The teacups are the vertebrae and the saucers are the discs in between the vertebrae. Any misalignment in that tall stack of dishes puts the entire structure at risk. The other force acting constantly on the human spine is gravity. Over time, gravity takes a tremendous toll even on a healthy spine. With my back curvature, I was even more in jeopardy. The almost daily nagging pain that plagued me was the main staple of my day. But after the car accident, matters were just amplified. It took several months of therapy and chiropractic care to get my soreness and aches down to a manageable level.

I kept up my physical activity with lawn care and play a fair amount of racquetball. Cutting lawns enabled me to make a few dollars while contemplating how to approach my educational future. My father was always a big advocate of a college education. He would repeatedly say, "No one can ever take an education away from you". I knew at this point I was going to re-focus on a doctorate in chiropractic.

In the fall that year, I enrolled in a small 2-year college in Dunwoody, Georgia in order to start on my journey. I remember a bit of intimidation on my first beginning days back at college. I went to school for a couple semesters, but did not fair too well. My grades were poor, so I decided to take a semester off and regroup. At that time, my lawn mowing business was taking off. I just focused on that endeavor.

What I enjoyed the most about the lawn care business, was that I enjoyed working outside, I was physically moving all the time, and the pay was worth the energy expended. This business was a good experience for me. I really grew as a person and a businessman. This was the beginning to my realization that self-employment was the way for me. No one person controlled my financial destiny. I built the business up to a certain point that I could handle. Needless to say, I was getting plenty of exercise.

WHERE DOES THE FIGHT COME FROM?

My scoliosis condition gave me a daily dose of pain and discomfort, usually in the mornings upon getting up.

As soon as I got up and took on the day, the back pain subsided. After a semester or two off from school and playing racquetball in the evenings, I came to the conclusion that I better get back into school; I didn't want to maintain lawns for the rest of my life.... becoming a doctor became the focus once again.

I commenced classes that following semester at the same college. With a refocused attitude and clearer mind, I attacked school. By this time all aspects of my life were going well. I was working hard for my lawn business, going to school, playing racquetball, traveling to racquetball tournaments. It felt like I was on some sort of autopilot. I even went over and took a tour of Life Chiropractic College in Marietta, Georgia; this just added more fuel to my fire to succeed.

This next event that I experienced was one of the top memorable moments in my adult life. My mother asked me one day if I would like to go see the surgeon that removed the Neuroblastoma from my body as a baby. Not realizing at the time the significance of it, I was not too excited with the idea. To me, it was another doctor from my past. In my mind, it was not in my best interest to revisit my past medical experience. I honored my mother's wishes and committed to go meet this man…this man who saved my life.

A week or so later, my mother and I went down near Emory Hospital, to an office park off of highway 85. I had mixed emotions in my head while riding down there to meet Dr. Gerald Zwiren. My thoughts were a whirlwind of my experiences. What would I say to this man besides 'thank you'? How would I react? How is one expected to react to such a situation? We walked into a modest, well-lit office into a waiting area with a frosted glass window on the other end of the reception area. I went to the window and was greeted and asked to sign in. When I turned around to sit down and wait to be called, I decided to have a look around. Upon glancing around the waiting room, I soon realized that this was not the routine sterile doctors office I had experienced in the past. All of the walls were covered with letters and attached photos of children. I walked around and read a few during my wait to see the man mentioned in each letter I read. As the sun beamed through the numerous glass windows, it did not take me long to shed my uneasy feelings of visiting this place. My eyes began to well up as I visited and read each letter. These letters were from children and young adults personally thanking the doctor for saving them or their brother or sister. They were written in crayon, colored pencil, and ink; some had photos; each letter told a story. It was very moving to see this type of display. What a reward for a doctor with a prestigious career. I pointed these letters out to my mother...she seemed content and quiet as if going through her own storm of memories from the corridors of her mind. It is still hard for me the fathom what my father and her dealt with regards to me.

The door opened to a hallway and a nurse called my name to invite me back. I proceeded down a hall to an exam room. She told me it was a pleasure to meet me and that the doctor has been waiting anxiously for your arrival. I thought it kind of strange at the time. Why would any doctor be anxious to see me? What made me special?

I waited a few minutes for Dr. Zwiren to come in the room. It was during that waiting period that I realized I did not know what this man looked like or would he really remember me.

When the door opened, in walked Dr. Zwiren in a white medical coat inscribed with his name and file in his hand. He called out my name "Bradley Dean Schmidt, How are you?" he said from across the room, "I am well and it is great to meet you". I remember I extended my hand for a handshake; he grabbed my hand to shake and moved to embrace me with a hug. I was a bit taken back at that moment for I had never really *met* this man. I had no memory of him. I was only told of his role in saving my life. He told me it was an honor to see me, I looked at him as his eyes were welled up.

For the next thirty minutes or so, we discussed my cancer, my surgeries and my medical history. He asked me how I felt, how difficult was it for me to move, stretch and bend. He had the look of amazement on his face as I gave him my explanation of myself. He took notes on all that I was saying as if he could not write fast enough. He asked me if I would mind taking my shirt off so that he could examine my back and my scars; I complied. While he examined me he was quiet. He ran his hands over my spine and next to my scars, examining them as if he were a sculptor examining his work. He said I looked fantastic. He raised a few questions about my ability to move; I told him I don't have any residual problems with movement or breathing in regards to my current condition. I told him I was playing a good bit of racquetball and mowing lawns. I felt good in telling him that because for most of my life the doctors who treated me did not recommend too much physical activity. I proved them wrong, I was in great shape for doing the opposite of their advice.

Upon finishing his examination, he asked me if I was uncomfortable with the way my backed appeared. He was referring to the sunken depression next to my lumbar spine where the tumor was removed. He mentioned his son; Dr. Jeffery Zwiren was a brilliant plastic surgeon. He could refer me over to him for an evaluation if I would like. I politely declined. In my mind I was determined not to ever go under the knife again. My mindset was if I had made it this far with the parts and conditions of my body; why jeopardize anything. If it was not broke, why take it apart and fix it. We both had a laugh with that analogy.

Dr Zwiren was just full of compliments and showered me with his joy that he radiated in his demeanor. He had such a warm presence in our discussion, very easy to talk to, as he genuinely listened to me.

He informed me that I was one of his most memorable patients of his long career. I felt bad that I had such a negative attitude on the way to see this man......*This is the man who saved my life; who gave me a chance!*

He asked me was I still planning on becoming a chiropractor. How he knew that, I was puzzled. Yes, I explained. He just agreed that was the good choice for me. He stopped and told me to wait here; he had something he wanted to show me. He left the room for few minutes while I got dressed from completing his examination. He came back a few moments later with a big file. Before he showed me the contents of the file, he informed me that my mother had periodically kept in contact with him after all these years. He knew about all my triumphs and progressions of the past two decades. He was so enamored with my case that he informed me that he had used the success of my case in his publications, teachings, and case studies. He seemed so very proud of me.

He glorified the fact that I survived the surgeries; I learned how to walk, and later run which was a tremendous accomplishment in itself. I was free of all braces, and to top it off the cancer had never returned. I asked him what he thought my odds were for survival. He exclaimed he did not think in odds; he just did what he thought he knew he could do. If he had to put it in odds... my odds were something like 1 in 100,000 of survival.

Dr. Zwiren expressed to me that my case was one of the most difficult cases to approach for him as a young surgeon. All of this was very overwhelming for me; to have someone explain to you how close to death you were. One thing he did tell me that he had informed my parents that I might not survive the second operation due to the invasiveness of the procedure. He felt it was the realistic thing to say to my parents at the time. "I had to prepare them for that possibility".

Upon completing the surgery and stitching me up, he had serious doubts that my body would endure through the night. He stated that when he returned to the hospital early that next morning, he ran down to intensive care to check on my status. " Your little heart monitor was still beeping; it was at that point, I knew you were going to make it....you were a "little fighter", and look at you now!". He then just embraced me.

We concluded our visit and he walked me out, as he did not know my mother accompanied me to his office. Upon seeing her, he extended his arms to embrace her. He greeted my mother like an old friend. He continued his praises of me, as our visit came to a close.

On the ride back home, my mother and I discussed my surgeries and treatments and relived it all again. Reflecting back in my life from today's point of view, meeting the man responsible for my existence on this earth was one of the top enlightening experiences of my life. In completing my research for this book, I discovered that Dr. Gerald T. Zwiren had passed away in 2002. I did, however, contact his son, Dr. Jeffery in 2010 and introduce myself to him. In a way, I just wanted one more chance to thank Dr. Gerald for the chance to be his patient. Dr. Jeffery informed me that his father had passed away in 2002 and that he lived a long passionate live; cases like mine were a reward of a long prestigious medical career. Dr. Jeff thanked me for contacting him and wished me much success with my book.

"Somewhere along the way...

I found a meaning."

~Joe Walsh

CHAPTER 9:
COLLEGE LIFE AND GRADUATION

After my meeting with Dr. Gerald Zwiren, it was safe to say, I did not lack the motivation and mind-set to move forward with my plans for college. By the fall of 1991, I finished most of the required classes to get accepted into Life College of Chiropractic in Marietta, Georgia. I spent most of the following year completing the necessary science classes in order to graduate into the doctorate program.

All this time I was working on classes; I continued to work in the lawn care business, as well as concentrate on racquetball tournaments. The class load I was attempting to complete at that point allowed me to work and play racquetball in the afternoons. Having a girlfriend became a focus of my attention as well. I recall that my grades were mainly (B's) and (C's) with the occasional (A). My focus was never on the grade; it was on what I got out of the class. Grades were of little importance to me other than a mark of completion. A mark of (F) meant that I had to take the class again, and out of initial frustration, I did until I received a passing grade. This occurred several times in my undergraduate college career.

At the time, I did not realize that not passing a class was a character builder, but in retrospect I became more focused. The important thing was to not give up; just keep moving forward.

After completing the requirements from the Life College School of Undergraduate Studies in the fall of 1992, I received a letter of Christmas break of my acceptance into the Doctor of Chiropractic Program. With a feeling of accomplishment of getting through some difficult classes, the holidays that year were a well-deserved break.

The following January 1993, I found myself starting my first quarter of the Doctor of Chiropractic program. Others had already warned me that the curriculum of classes coming at me would be difficult, stressful, and unfair, along with other descriptions. After attending the orientation, I was very intimidated. They tell you that so many of you are starting, but only a few of you will finish. The first year of chiropractic school was a weeding out process. The first year was not easy for me; I struggled with classes right away. It was such a tremendous amount of information coming at you at an incredible rate that this became the challenge just to pass the class. Many of the classes were built on the previous class. So if you did not pass class (A), then you could not continue to class (B). This relationship of classes always instilled fear to pass everything that curriculum demanded.

I had my struggles right way when starting the program. Racquetball soon became a low priority in my life; my evenings and weekends were soon spent trying to study and process all that was coming at me. Having a girlfriend was just out of the question; there was just limited time. I seemed to expand on an intellectual level during this time. Time management became the main concern for me. Getting the most out of the waking hour was the goal of the day. I would travel to school for a 7AM class and stay on campus until my classes were done. Then I would leave the campus and go and cut three or four lawns, and then go home to shower and eat, and then head to a bookstore to study. I was trying to cut 25 or so lawns a week and go to school. Looking back on this regiment, I do not know how I survived it. I just wanted to become a doctor so badly that I ignored what I was going through; just the end result of completing all these classes was my reinforcement. Time seemed to pass so quickly. Classes went by in a minute and soon it was Christmas again. In my opinion, you never know what you are capable of until you are put under pressure. The rate that information was coming at me was unbearable at times. I was making forward progress with the curriculum; that was the main agenda.

I remember at times I would almost fall under the pressure of the demands of a doctorate program. Dead-lines and tests just consumed me; I remember thinking to myself, 'I got to do this, I will complete this program....just get to the end and become a doctor'.

There was a period in school where students had to practice on each other the art of palpation, which is just simple examining the body and getting to know the structure of the spine through touch.

I was very reluctant to have any of my fellow student practice on me as my spine was in such a disorder with regards to scoliosis. Eventually, I overcame this shyness and allowed instructors and student to examine me. Of course each new group of classes meant that I had to explain myself over and over again.

About the second year of classes I started Human Anatomy Class and Dissection Lab. I knew this was coming at me with the schedule of classes. I feel I have to describe this event to you, as it was one of the unique experiences of my life. This is the class made of two parts where the student gets to dissect a real human body from head to toe, male and female. The first part focused on the dissection of the torso of a cadaver. The second part consisted of the arms, legs and head.

When I walked into that cadaver lab at 7am, I felt like a soldier reporting for boot camp. Upon entering the lab, I was greeted with the view of 8 to 10 body bags lying on dissection tables.

WHERE DOES THE FIGHT COME FROM?

As students, nothing prepares you enough to see that sight. The first thing that hits you upon entering the cold lab is the smell of formaldehyde. This is a smell that I never will forget. It is a pungent smell that immediately starts to irritate your senses. I remember glancing around looking at all the other 'virgins' in here with their fresh white lab coats, dissection tools, as well as extra rubber gloves; they all had blank stairs on their faces as the anatomy instructor read our names off of a roll sheet and continued on with the instructional protocol of the lab.

We were given specific instructions on how we were to conduct ourselves in dealing with bodies donated to the betterment of science. The instructor handed us a packet with a list of all the structure we would be tested on the midterm and final; just two exams. The packet was like a small phone book. I flipped through the packet with over 1500 structures to identify and name for the course. I remember a feeling of uneasiness came about me. By the next hour, we gathered around a body bag in the center of the room as instructed. We were advised that if anyone had a problem viewing or dissecting a human body, they could request what they call "dry lab". This is where the student could view just plastic models. All the students looked at each other as to see who would opt out for dry lab first....who would be the weakest link?

When the removal of the body from the body bag was complete, the body was then unwrapped. The head, hands, feet, and sexual organs were left covered. This was the first time I had seen an actual deceased human body in a lab setting. This particular body was male; I would guess in his late 70's. I remember just staring in a comatose manner at this specimen. The instructor stated we would spend this first week of lab just observing him doing the initial cutting on the body in order to display to us how to conduct a proper dissection.

I recall when the initial cutting started with the lab instructor and his assistant; a few people had to leave. It was as if they left to go use the restroom and never came back. I did not see them again for the rest of the course. I will not go into the rest of what I saw and did while taking the Anatomy Labs for the doctorate program.

A statement I can say is that over time I worked on several bodies, I reached higher awareness to the fact that the human body is amazing machine.

When I became a patient in student clinic, I had to be x-rayed. When the staff, instructors and fellow students viewed them; they would gather around the x-ray view box as if they were viewing an alien for the first time. Doctors would summon other doctors to see the x-rays as well. With this gathering, came a barrage of questions.

These kinds of occasions were my first steps in getting use to talking about my condition in public.

When it came to the point in my chiropractic curriculum where I would learn spinal adjustments, reluctance came over me. I just became uncomfortable with anyone working on me. They would say, "How do you move with a spine in this condition?" My spine looked like an "S" with its curves and positions. I responded with, ' I do not know how I move and walk; I ignore the pain of scoliosis and just move. My body has some how adapted to the condition.' Some would say that I was on many levels a miracle. Call it what you want...I am just here doing what I do.

Through out my experience at Life Chiropractic College there were a few instructors who lashed out in their teachings about the medical profession. I found this very offensive at first, and then I realized they expressed a dissent for the medical profession in order to further their point of view. I always said to myself, if it was not for the numerous doctors, nurses and specialist...I would not be sitting in this class right now. Instructors who portrayed the medical profession as a demonic monster, were not worth my time, therefore, instead of disputing with them, I elected to transfer to another section. In some cases, I would just do the bare minimum to pass the class and move on.

CHAPTER 9: COLLEGE LIFE AND GRADUATION

I remember one assignment I had to write a paper about chiropractic care and its benefits. I wrote the paper about my life, and surviving cancer; including some chiropractic care. This was one of those headstrong instructors who spoke of chiropractic as the cure for every condition; the medical profession was a lost group of people providing nothing to the sick. The day came when we got our papers back in class; I received a grade of "D". Needless to say, I was fuming mad. I walked up to the instructor and asked to speak to him during his office hours; he agreed. The following morning, I went to his office. He asked my why I was there; I stated I was upset with him about the grade I received. I showed him my paper; as he looked it over, I glanced around his cluttered small office, with chiropractic paraphernalia on every square inch of his walls. This guy was a Doctor of Chiropractic; I thought to myself that surely my grade was some sort of mistake. He looked it for a brief time and then handed it back to me as if he was throwing it away a dirty napkin. He said I lacked chiropractic focus in the paper. I stated that I simply told my story; but in that story, the medical profession was the focus. Chiropractic care was only the ladder part of my experience. I was very upset with this and decided to take this matter to the Dean, which I did. Before I left the instructor's office, I turned around upon exiting and said I think that you made a mistake with this grade, and realize one thing….'You have the *luxury* of not knowing what I know'. I left it at that. I went to the Dean; he was no help either. I decided to drop the class and take it again with a different instructor. Incidents like this were common for me in college. I realize now that they helped build my character. These types of situation educated me on how to deal with problems and problematic people. Over six years passed in order to obtain a doctorate degree. I went into Chiropractic College as a naive, unaware individual. I came out a confident, motivated and focused person. In retrospect, my college experience made me a man.

It was during the ladder part of school that I went to work for a chiropractor that I had met at a local racquetball tournament. I started playing again after a four-year break due to school. It was there I learned how to run an office, deal with patients, take x-rays, and adjust patients with different techniques. This was a growth period for me as well as a time for mental maturity; I enjoyed it. I could not wait to get out in the real world and work as a Chiropractor.

What and experience it was to graduate as a Doctor of Chiropractic in December 1999. I participated in a Commencement Ceremony a few months before my actual graduation with my parents in attendance. It was a tremendous experience for me. I knew my parents were proud of me as I experienced all of this. With all the struggles I have endured, this was the fruit of my labor. I remember I had to go to an Exit Interview in December 1999, in order to be released from school; this is where they go over your records to make sure all is in order.

This interview took about an hour with a doctor from the Dean's office doing the scrutinizing of your records. I finished the interview and was congratulated; I shook hands and with my college records in my hand, the interview ended. When I walk out of that interview, I exited the administration building and headed for my car, which was illegally parked; I did this out of defiance. My thought was it was my last visit to the campus; what are they going to do to me? I got in my car and just sat there and wept. I had completed Chiropractic School...I was a doctor. When I got my diplomas a month or so later just reinforced a feeling of satisfaction that I had completed something great. I had all of them framed and hanging in our home; I view them daily as a constant reminder of personal achievement. I remember way back to the beginning of college and thinking of getting a doctorate....what a long road; *but I did it* and *I knew I could* !

After graduation, I focused on moving into a new apartment with a girl I was dating while changing my behavior from that of a student to a working adult. Completing graduate school was comparable to getting off of a huge roller coaster ride. Going from fast pace, with dead-lines, tests, seeing patients in out patient clinic at school as well as other commitments; to just going to work and coming home, was an unusual shift.

Racquetball and working the lawn business took on more momentum since I was no longer a student. I imme-diately started working as many hours as I could at the chiropractic office, and on the off days working outside with lawn care. I was very driven at this time. My goal was to get licensed in chiropractic, develop a practice with doctor I was working with, and just advance from that level. I continued to increase my activity, and exposure with racquetball; I was playing four times a week or more. I started to get the fire to compete again. My girlfriend at the time unfortunately did not like me playing so much as I would get home late in the evening. I just said to her, I had to play in order to feel better.

I worked hard over the next two years at the clinic, working my chiropractic business, still kept my lawn business going as a back up income resource. I was at a point in my life where I was driven to succeed by my ego. I want to make as much money as I could as I had an up and coming lifestyle to support. We had moved to an even more exclusive apartment in a suburb of Atlanta near the chiropractic clinic. I wanted to get married and buy a home and start a family. I took me a while to realize during this time my life that I really was not making any headway on the success ladder. With the increases in lifestyle expenses and the struggles of starting a chiropractic career, the numbers were just not adding up.

Making money as a chiropractor even with a partner became ever increasingly difficult. It was at this time that most of my business was basically controlled by payments form the various insurance companies. I had to wait to get paid on patients whose insurance was there only payment option. When an insurance company begins to control the time line of payments as well as what they will pay; then a chiropractor gets put into a precarious position. The insurance company dictated how much you could see the patient as well. I began to fight and argue my position. Then who is the doctor in this relationship? Without a doubt, it was the insurance company.

I had had enough; I became disenchanted with the chiropractic business by that time. I became very disappointed with myself. I genuinely cared for the patient; I wanted to help all that I could. If I can't make a living at it, then I would have to make some decisions.

I felt like I had gone to school for such a large part of my adult life that how could I recover from this?

I then came up with the solution to get re-educated. I would attempt to go on to medical school and major in osteopathic medicine. Being that I was in that ego driven mind-set, I thought, take it to the next level. I went on to take the MCAT on two occasions and visit two medical schools. I broke up with the girlfriend at the time because she was not on the same sheet of music as myself. I found myself at a pivotal point in my life; what do I do?

I ended my chiropractic business abruptly in 2003 as well as ended several toxic relationships in my life in order to clear my plate and really reinvent myself. Some close friends of mine who now lived in Florida offered me a place to stay in order to get out of Atlanta, Georgia and clear my head. They lived in Tampa, not far from the beach. So in one week, I broke up with my girlfriend, cancelled my lease on my apartment, moved all my stuff into storage, and drove to Tampa for a new chapter to begin.

"Keep on going and chances are you will stumble into something...I have never heard of anyone stumbling on something sitting down."

~Charles F. Kettering

CHAPTER 10:
REINVENTING MYSELF

I moved to Florida to do a little soul searching. Upon relocating to North Tampa in the fall of 2003, all I wanted was fresh start, some time off from life, and just work on reinventing myself. I lived in a beautiful home in an affluent community called Tampa Palms. I spent the next few months basically relaxing, playing racquetball, working on my tan, fishing with friends; it was a good time. I met a few quality people during this time.

I did remember at some point I had to really question myself in regards to what do I want to do with my life. I had stayed in touch with several friends back in Atlanta, one of whom was an attorney who I knew from playing racquetball. John was the attorney I had met at the courts on evening. We had met at the courts one evening, not knowing each other's occupation. We quickly became friends. As soon as we disclosed what we did for a living, our friendship grew even stronger. It was hard to disengage form the chiropractic business for me. I did not look at it as a failure; I just looked at it as the result of a non-success.

When I moved away, I stayed in touch with John for some reason. He has tenaciousness and perseverance that I admired. I confided in him with sharing the story of my distaste for the education choice that I made. He was a tremendous help at that time when I needed it the most; he helped me in humorous way. There was always a joke at the end of his logic. I think looking back, what I admired was that he was genuine. This is a quality that is hard to find in people today. As an example.... I am of German descent, and John is of Jewish decent. Our backgrounds have never come between our relationship. We always joke with each other back and forth about our backgrounds with mutual respect.

After staying in Tampa for almost a year, I soon realized that I had better focus in on what I wanted to do with my life. I knew I had to move back to Atlanta at some point, to be with my family and to start in a new direction. I moved back to Atlanta in 2004. I immediately wanted to restart my lawn business as well as reengage into the racquetball community. Staying in touch with John in the interim, turn out to be a blessing in disguise.

I resumed playing racquetball with my usual group or guys, including John. On one occasion, John was in a rush to leave the courts for several appointments he had with his potential clients. He had too many clients coming at him at once; he therefore asked me if I would go interview them, as they were personal injury clients from auto accidents. I agreed and then met him at his office the following week to be instructed on how to interview potential clients. I then went out and met these new clients, documented their injuries, had them sign papers to get legal representation, and returned to the law firm. Within a short period of time, I was a busy man. I began to work for John more and more as time passed. My schedule was very flexible; it still allowed for my other endeavors.

I kept on with my lawn business, and playing racquetball as well as tournaments. I lived with my family at this time in my life. I was still trying to figure out which direction to head. For now, I had several jobs and living arrangements were met. Over the year, I decided to try to get into medical school for a degree in Osteopathic Medicine. As I stated before, ended up taking the MCAT twice. I scored marginally as most people do when they take this sort of test.

I looked at two different schools, one in Georgia, and the other in Florida. With my workload at the law firm increasing, I decided that I was going to stay in Atlanta and work that program for a while. I liked the schedule of the job. I could schedule my own appointments once the case was referred to me. It allowed me such a freedom that I soon realized was a valuable thing. There is a certain satisfaction to basically being your own boss. You only have a finite allotment of time each day; how you spent the time is important for the quality of one's life.

Since my graduation from grad school, my ego had been driving my direction. During this time of soul searching, I was exposed to a tape that a friend gave me. On that tape was a recording of a speech by Dr Wayne Dyer. He is a self-help professional. On that tape there were some insightful thoughts and stories about trying to find you path in life. One of the main ideas of the speech was that an individual's happiness is generated from within that individual. There is no outside source of happiness. He stated so many people today are looking in other places; clubs, religion, work, in others, etc. in order to find happiness.

This insightful perspective struck a cord with me. I soon realized that I was on a path that was dictated by my ego. At that point, I decided to let go of my ego and my desire to succeed in a material way. I had to let go of worry and disappointment with where my life had taken me. I decided that going back to school was maybe not in my best interest. I put that idea on suspension and focused on my work with the attorney. I enjoyed the work most of the time. I got to meet all kinds of people from all walks of life. I made my own hours, and scheduled my time according-ly. I expanded my services to include other law firms while still keeping a small lawn business going. By 2005, I had bought my first home in a suburb of Atlanta. I worked diligently for the next two years, with the focus mainly on the intent for self-improvement. I was on a quest at that time to rediscover who I really was. I remember getting heavy into reading, mainly on topics of spirituality, self-discovery, and enlightenment. I shifted my habits of what I read, what I watched, to what music I listen to. I got away from the mainstream.

Once I disconnected from the mainstream, including watching television, my mind cleared out and became calmer and more as ease. I was able to focus more clearly. I still had many unanswered questions in my mind as in the direction I needed to head in order for self-satisfaction. You tend to really examine your life once all the noise is taken out of it. I came to the rational that I had many reasons to be thankful. Possessing many tools and abilities, my focus became choosing a direction to set sail.

CHAPTER 11:
LIFE WITH MY NEW BRIDE

The next chapter that happened to me was an event that altered the path of my life. A few months prior to this event, I had all but given up on meeting the right woman. I had not had much success in the past with meeting a suitable partner for a life-long relationship. With frustration at its peak, I chose to discontinued trying to pursue. My shift in attention just went to training for tournaments, working, and spending time with friends and family. I had complete confidence with being by myself.

One of my very good friends, Dr. Tim Hansen, asked me to play in a doubles racquetball tournament in which I initially turned down. When he told me he already registered us for the event, I then agreed. Reluctantly, I went to the tournament. However, I was glad to be playing in the event with such high-ranking player. We shared a common link, as he was one of my classmates from Life Chiropractic College. I walked into the racquetball club just a few minutes before our match. To arrive just before my match was common for me, as I like to just walk on and play. I don't like to arrive early and talk to everyone before a match as it takes away from my focus for being there…..*to win*. Upon entering the facility, I walked through a foyer crowded with people. With my head down and walking at a pace so that I don't make contact with anyone, I headed to the registration desk to pay my entry fee. There was a small line there of people there waiting as well. Taking my wallet out from my bag and getting my things in order…that was when I saw her.

She was working at the registration desk taking in the checks and registering the players for the event. She was absolutely breath taking in my opinion. As the line diminished, it became my turn.

She had such natural beauty about her; I recall a feeling of nervousness came about me. Half way through the transaction, I thought to myself, 'Introduce yourself to her'. So I extended my hand to her and did so.

The moment I took her hand and she told me her name, I had a strange feeling. She said her name was Allison. I told her I had to play but I would be back to talk to her. I thought to myself, a woman who possesses this amount of beauty and grace would most likely be in a relationship. Once my racquetball match started in a glass court near the front desk where Allison was working, I found it difficult to concentrate on the match at hand; my mind was in another place. Thanks to the abilities of my partner Tim, we were triumphant. With so much anticipation, I could not wait to go back up and talk to her. It turns out during the match a friend of mine had gone up to

Allison and informed her that I was interested in her. I expressed my interest for her before I walked on the court. A friend of mine over heard me and approached her. This was the start of her interest in me. I had my doubts that a girl this attractive and beautiful, who handled herself with such an effortless grace, would be single herself.

After several conversations that day, it turns out that she was single. She had been single for several months, as she had become disenchanted with her last relationship. I could not believe this information. I left the tournament that evening with the anticipation of seeing her on the following day. The following day arrived, after continued conversations that day, I asked her if she would like to have lunch with me the following weekend; she agreed. I remember we talked for several hours during the week prior to our first date. Just from our conversations, I knew she was special. I did not initially tell her about my battle with cancer as I thought it would be overwhelming.

We went out that following weekend; and the rest was history. With our relationship budding, we were together as much as we time allowed during the week as she commuted to school from her family's home. The time came when I felt it was appropriate to let her know my story about my operations, cancer, scoliosis and learning to play racquetball. She hugged me and held me close as I concluded my story. Being a little nervous that she would reject me on that level; she did not. We dated for several months, just spending as much of our evenings together as our schedules would allow. She was a collegiate runner for a state school in Georgia, so we had a lot in common as far as being athletic; this was one of our common denominators.

We had both been hurt in past relationships; as well as decided to be single and focus on our own situation rather than randomly date. It turns out, after several months of dating, we were meant to be together. We started spending more and more free time together until several months later we moved in together. Allison and I were finally happy. Our lives in such a way that we just blended together. I began to feel more complete knowing that I had a beautiful, focused, and motivated young lady at my side. As well as she found comfort and support with me at her side. Over the next year, our lives evolved and changed as we became more solid in our relationship. It is in my opinion that you should spend at least a year getting to know someone before you escalate the relationship.

We were engaged in February 2009 in Tybee Island, Georgia. I asked here to marry me while walking on the beach in the early evening. I had never been so nervous. I hid the ring in a shell and placed it on the ground near us as we were collecting shells before sunset. I hid it in the seaweed when she was not looking, as we were walking near the pier. I pointed to a clamshell, which was closed, in the seaweed. I told her to collect it. She would not pick it up for fear that there was something in it still alive. I picked up the shell and reassured her that it was ok to open the shell…..she did! With a quiet voice, I asked her to marry me…and the answer was yes! We just held each other as tears welled up in our eyes; we both were just overjoyed!

In a slow pace and holding hands, we strolled down the beach back to the hotel. Allison and I would stop walking and just embrace each other and kiss….these are the great moments in life. I just did not want to end that walk on the beach before sunset. She was anxious to get back to the hotel and share the news with her family.

With the sound of the ocean, the warm sand under our feet, and the sea gulls flying over our heads, we walked hand in hand back towards the hotel, stopping briefly to look at the ring….and embrace each other.

We were married in October of 2009, in Tybee Island, with a few family and friends present. The ceremony took place in the afternoon out on the beach in the dunes. It was a cool, windy day; I remember that the sun was out and I was experiencing such as sense of joy. Here I was, experiencing a moment I honestly thought I would never reach. Allison's family came down for the weekend to attend the wedding.

WHERE DOES THE FIGHT COME FROM?

With my mother, father, and brothers as witnesses, we were married on that cool October afternoon in a simple ceremony in the dunes. When the minister said, "I now pronounce you man and wife", a feeling of joy and exhilaration came over me. I did not feel the cool wind blowing around me; it was as if a feeling of calmness and relaxation.

To be truthful, I never thought I would find a woman like Allison. She continues to be, one of the great experiences of my life. I planned on getting married just once in my life; I had made my mind up with that idea. I had waited many years to find the right woman to share my life with, which made the experience of getting married even that more special for me. Many doubts played through my mind in the sense that would a girl ever want to marry me. My body was not complete, and I was physically scared from my surgeries.

When I finally shared my life story with her a few weeks after we met, she later told me that my story moved her in such a way that her bond with me grew even stronger. I thought my history with cancer and scoliosis would scare her away from me; but I was wrong. With our common likes and dislikes and competitive spirit, we have formed a solid long-lasting relationship. She supports me in all my endeavors as I support her. We enjoy the simple things in life, as we share each day that goes by. It is a great feeling for me during racquetball matches at tournaments to look out and see her watching me play, cheering me on, and smiling because I won a rally; she tells me "I am your number one fan". On many occasions, I stop and think of all the events that transpired; how long it took us to meet, how we met, and the life that we now share. I am simply overjoyed with how these events fell into place and altered the path my life.

To live is the rarest thing in the
world....Most people just exist,
and that's all."
~Oscar Wilde

CHAPTER 12:
REALIZING MY PURPOSE

With my new bride at my side, Allison and I embarked on our married lives together. With a solid foundation together we returned to Atlanta the following week of the wedding rested and recharged, ready to further plan our future. I immediately refocused on increasing my workload while spending as much time with my wife. As with life, a turn of events brought me an unfortunate circumstance that increased my awareness that I need to share my story about my cancer.

In 2008, I found out that one of my racquetball friends just diagnosed. His name was David; we were racquetball acquaintances. David was just a couple years younger than myself; he was in the prime of his life. He was in his late 30's; married, successful, athletic; and great racquetball player. A mutual friend of ours called me with a 'Did you hear the news?' type of call; David has cancer. It was the type of call that made me feel so hurt; this news could not be true. I saw David a month or so prior to this devastating news. David knew I was a cancer survivor; I just had to talk to him.

I immediately called him and left him a message to call me, as I was concerned about him. He called me back; he informed me with the news a person doesn't want to hear. I pulled over into a parking lot in order to talk. We ended up talking for almost 2 hours. He informed me that he had Malignant Melanoma; I was so taken back by this, as he was a little matter of fact about his situation. He knew about my battles with cancer and the aftermath; I think he just confided in me.

All I could tell him that it was just a diagnosis; you give it power and meaning on your own behalf. The news of all this took a while to mentally sink in for him. We talked a couple time a week from that point after as he went in for the menagerie of tests and evaluations to check the progression and location of this devastating type of cancer. Metastatic Melanoma is very invasive and aggressive by nature; I just told David to focus on trying to survive this ordeal.

We met for lunch a few weeks later after one of his doctor appointments. He shared with me with all the sad statistics the medical profession informed him were the odds in this game of survival. He talked to me as if he was already programmed to loose this war before the battle had really begun.

Over and over again, I told him to ignore the statistics; I didn't want to hear them. I did not want to hear the statistic because I felt a non-belief in statistics and cancer. At one point, he stopped and asked me, 'What would you do if you were me? What medical path would you take? I paused for a moment as to carefully think about my response as to not to offend him.

He stated to that it was hard to figure out which direction to take as he felt he was in great condition; the diagnosis of cancer had not made him feel physically different. It was just hard to accept the diagnosis. "Then don't accept it; go on living your life. But also, change your life." What I meant by this was to stop in your tracks, and evaluate *exactly* what you are doing to your body on a daily basis. Ask yourself, is what I am putting in my body good for the body as a whole? Ask yourself, am I getting enough exercise and rest. I was not saying that you could go home and sit on a yoga mat, take some vitamins, drink some water, light a candle, and hum this cancer away.

I informed him that "wellness" is the lifestyle that I base my activities around. My lifestyle is both mental and physical. I told him my thoughts about his situation; how to proceed cautiously and make educated decisions for future medical care. It is in my opinion that a fear came over him at some point in his experience with all of this. We would talk on the phone every few weeks and he would tell me what the doctors and nurses had said. David had set up a blog on the internet to give people who were trying to contact him an update on his condition without getting on the phone and having to repeat himself 20 times a day.

As the blog evolved over the late summer and fall of 2008, I could read the frustration and mental breakdown; his cancer was progressing at a high rate. The doctors wanted to try one more test, one more drug, one more scan; he became disenchanted with it all. He even began to question God. It was very difficult for me to read his blog as his writing style became less informative and more based on anger. It was very understandable at the time the reasons for his frustration, for he was in uncharted seas. With no concrete answers or solutions, many battles with cancer end in this manner. My last conversation with him was a few weeks before he passed away. David was heading to his parents farm to spend time there and rest. I told him to go be alone on his family property. Go walk in nature, go fishing alone, go hiking, be by yourself and think.

I mentioned to him that we should get together for a meal and catch up when he returns. About three weeks after that call, I tried to reach David on the phone to no avail. I left another week go by as I figured he was still at his parent's farm, which had limited phone service. He had no blog entries at this time. I became concerned when I called him twice on a weeknight and received no return call or email. In a later conversation with his wife, I was calling David on his phone during the moment he was passing on. Something inside of me told me to reach out and call him.

I received a call from a mutual friend the next day informing me that David had passed away the night before. I was devastated; I did not get to see my friend for the last time. It had taken less than a year for the cancer to take its toll on him. After going to the service and the funeral, I stayed after to talk to David's wife. I told her I was trying to reach him for the last couple weeks as I was getting concerned. She told me he came home from the farm and started feeling the affects of cancer and the treatments. He lost a good amount of weight in the last two weeks. With his hair spars and condition worsening, David decided to disconnect from everyone; he wanted to pass on in private...and he did.

David was a great friend; it was quite a loss for me. Stories like David's play out on a daily basis. His plight made me realize once again, how fortunate I am to have the gift of life. David's passing allowed me to re-examine my own existence. He changed my focus on the importance of realization of what is really relevant in life. I visit his grave from time to time to spend a moment with him, as I was not in his presence when he passed on. I "talk" to him and let him know about the goings on in my life. A feeling of peace comes over me when I leave the cemetery; it is just a good thing for me to do. I know that when I leave my visit with David, that I recondition and realign my mind. People think that going to a cemetery is a depressing or morbid thing to do. I disagree; I get uplifted and empowered. I become more aware of act of living and how it is all taken for granted. There is not any drug on the market that can do that for a person. Awareness and peace are the boundless feelings that I strive to magnify each day that I am here on this earth.

With this awareness and outlook on life, I started a new life together with my wife, Allison. I wanted to work even harder with all of my endeavors. However, while working harder, it was important for me to work smarter. I changed my work schedule in order to work more from home and decrease my time away from my wife. With this shift in place, my schedule could be dictated from a more efficient manner. The free time that was created allowed for a better quality of life.

All of these shifts in life style were the prelude to me authoring this book. The allotments of time that I created, allowed me to re-examine myself. I ended up getting up earlier in the day when things were calm; making coffee, and reading for an hour or so before the workday started. Over the next several months, this was my daily routine.

After a while, there were more instances along the way that aided me with the idea of publishing my story.

WHERE DOES THE FIGHT COME FROM?

Throughout my adult life, several people I have met who were informed about my life story, told me "You need to tell people your story". This was the statement that would resonate in my mind like the sound of a bell after it has been struck. That day my mother passed to me a box of my medical records and told me to keep these records, they will mean so much to you; was the pinnacle sign for me to put my story together. I meet all kinds of people within the legal profession and I see the challenges and struggles that people endure. They perceive minor issues as huge problems, complicated by choices they made in their lives; I find it amazing that some of these people function. I leave sometimes after meeting these types of people, thinking to myself, 'I don't have any problems; and I made some good choices in my life'.

There was actually a time in my life where I possessed an embarrassment about my cancer battle and scoliosis. Now as an adult, an attempting to figure out which direction to set sail in my life; I realize now that I have been carrying this great story of survival and perseverance around with me. It would be foolish for me to ignore what is right in front of me....I just did not see it; until now.

So early on mornings before sunrise I sat down at the computer and started compiling the information to construct my autobiography. After organizing medical records, doing phone interviews, and organizing all the photos and questioning family members; I started writing. Most of this book was written in the early morning hours of the day; when everything was calm. Almost a year later, I am writing the final chapter!

What better way to serve my fellow mankind than to give back with an inspiring story like this to pass on to someone that there is a way out of a difficult situation. I would hope to instill in people both young and old, that the body is an amazing and complex machine. It is a machine that was designed to adapt to its environment no matter what the conditions are at hand. If just one person read this story and became enlightened, changed their outlook on themselves; and altered their path to a more positive outcome; then it was worth it for me to share my life story…I would have succeeded.

In all my readings, the most moving author for me is Ralph Waldo Emerson. He has a great quote that basically exemplifies my feelings as I conclude this book and start on a new path in my life of helping people.

~ *"To laugh often and much, to win the respect and the affection of children, to earn the appreciation of honest critics and endure the betrayal of false friends, to appreciate beauty, to find the best in others, to leave the world a bit better, whether by a healthy child, a garden patch.....to know that one life has breathed easier because you have lived. This is to have succeeded!*

~ *Ralph Waldo Emerson*

"Never bend your head. Always hold it high. Look the world straight in the face."

~Helen Keller; speaking to a 5 year-old blind child

Conclusion: A New Direction

In conclusion to all of this, I want to thank so many people who were instrumental to me and continue to make up the fabric of my life.........

To my mother and father, there are just not enough words that I can express the gratitude and respect that they have exemplified through out my entire life. All that they have provided and given to me is a story within itself. They have been and continue to be the very foundation that defines me. I owe many thanks to my immediate family; who also helped me in so many different ways. The many doctors, nurses and other medical and chiropractic professionals who each played an intricate role in allowing me to get to this day as healthy individual; I could not praise you all enough. To my wife, whose love, caring, understanding, and support both inspires me and makes me aware of how special our union plays a role as we move forward with our lives. There have been many friends along the way, some who have had time cut short, and some that support me to this day; I say a special thanks to you all.

On May 28, 2010, I spoke via phone the Dr. Michael Levine of Northside Pediatrics, in Atlanta, Georgia. This is the man who first discovered and realized that a possible tumor was growing inside of me. I had called his office the day before and left his office manager a message to have Dr Levine call me. I told her that I was one of his old patients from the 1970's and that I was writing a book about my experience with cancer. Within the same day, Dr Levine had returned my call in the early evening. His message was one of excitement and well wishes. I was deeply moved to hear this voicemail from a man who I have not had interaction with over 35 years. Dr Michael Levine, as my childhood Pediatrician, was instrumental in referring my case to Dr Gerald Zwiren. My parents first took me to see him in the winter of 1968 after my family had just moved to Atlanta, Georgia. After almost 35 years had past since I had been his patient, I felt nervous to even call this man. In working on this book project, I felt it incumbent on me to contact all the instrumental people I could to make them aware of my tremendous gratitude and thanks for playing a key role in my journey to get to this day. Speaking to Dr. Levine was such an honor. His genuine compassion and caring for the patient just radiated through his voice. I felt a tremendous honor to tell him about my life in our brief conversation. He asked several questions about my well-being, my family, and if I was married. He told me that to hear from me after all this time, and after all that I had been through, can really make a physicians career. It is like the prize at the end of a long career in practice. He is now retired from practice and enjoying his golden years still residing in Atlanta, Georgia. He asked me to stay in touch with him, and to call him in the near future to get together to see each other. When I told him I was in the middle of a writing project compiling the story of my life...he said he would love to read it and share in its creation.

We both met at a coffee shop on May 6th, 2011. I arrived a half hour early to compose myself for I felt a tremendous honor in meeting this man who was so important in this story. Dr Levine came walking up to me in the shop and greeted me like an "old friend". We talked and shared stories of our personal lives over the course of our meeting. He was so complementary in his statements.

He thought it was great that my life's path has brought this book to reality. The world needs to hear more stories like mine, he exclaimed. After a 45-minute meeting with him, we said our goodbyes and promised to keep in touch. I had a customer in the shop take a photo us for posterity. I left our meeting feeling so enlightened, for meeting him, was yet another great reward in my life.

I wake up each day, especially after bringing this writing project to a conclusion, with a greater appreciation of the frailty of life. This past year has really been an introspective time in my life where I can really stop and examine my experiences. I am traveling down the long hallway of life with many doors on either side, as I discussed in the beginning of this book. Some of the doors I have opened were detrimental to me but many of the doors have led to great people and experiences.

Now, as a grown adult, I can confidently stop in my steps and look back down that long hallway of life and say that I made it through all that, and I appreciated into a better person. I use appreciated in the sense that I feel that I have increased in value as a person; *I am just better than I use to be.*

I think that my fight, will to survive and ability to overcome obstacles came from an innate power within me. It is some phenomenon that came with me being born. Each positive outcome in the past has built my confidence and outlook to a point where I was not going to give up on the task at hand until I see the desired result.

It all seem mysterious to me………

I notice that a shift has taken place in my life, especially in the past two years. Now that I am married, an evolution to calm has taken place. I have evolved into a quiet, observer type individual.

My attention now is to enjoy more peace in my life. The times at the beach in the early morning when it is just myself walking on the beach with just the sound of the ocean and sea gulls. I cherish those moments, as there are invaluable. Enjoying times with my wife, family and close friends have also become cherished.

I have reduced and also refused to clutter my life with all the groups, clubs, agendas that come my way on a daily basis. In society today, there is too much focus on what 'group' you belong to. The group is disguised as religious, employer, sports team, schools, the list goes on an on. My thought is that once you give your attentions over to a group, you forfeit your individual spirit and self-reliance. We are today, so focused on this aspect of belonging to a group. I see it in my travels; the advertising, the bumper stickers, and in the discussions of the people I meet.

I have never claimed to be better than anyone else on this planet. But there are times when I do realize that I am amazed that the chapters of my life played out as they did. A higher level of awareness has become the product of the sum of my experiences. It is my thought that if people could shift there thinking less on group issues and more on personal development, maybe the interactions of people would be less problematic.

From time to time I do have a chance to meet a person who has been through a horrific experience like cancer, or medical condition, or an accident of some kind. The common outcome of that experience is an increased awareness and appreciation of life. I often wonder to myself that ' It would be a invaluable teaching to be taught this level of personal awareness at a young age'. Why does one have to go through a challenging experience to become enlightened? It is impossible to pass this awareness on to another who has not directly experienced what one has been through. It is like teaching another person how to swim who has never been in the water. You can tell them how to move their arms and legs and swim; they may *believe* they can swim. They will never *know* how to swim, until they themselves venture into the water.

It is my view now that life is not a dress rehearsal for a monumental event in one's life. I am aware that I all I have is today…and the hope of tomorrow! Enjoyment of each day is the mantra that I try to exemplify. Living in the simple mindset has allowed me to enjoy more of the daily experiences that come my way. When I walk with my wife and our dogs in the woods, I take in all nature displays to me. The sounds, the smell, the flowers, the birds….it is all amplified to me. I say a silent 'thank you' to the powers that be with a feeling of appreciation and gratitude as I take it all in.

There have been times I have experienced a new type of pain of discomfort in my body related to my scoliosis. I have asked myself, 'What is that pain; is cancer coming back?' In the next thought I would say to myself…**'absolutely not**!!' I have lived this long; there is a reason and purpose for me. I brush off the negative thoughts as soon as they have come up.

With the lifestyle that I now lead; proper exercise, diet, conditioning, and positive thinking, there is no reason not to live a prosperous and peaceful life. I still to this day, play racquetball as much as six times a week to stay active. That sport has given me freedom. Freedom from braces, freedom from surgery, freedom from a wheelchair, and most importantly, the freedom of mobility.

There are certain rules that I abide by in life. I have limited the amount of processed foods, no fast foods, and no sodas. I enjoy tea, coffee, wine and water. I am insanely active with exercise. I do not smoke cigarettes or use drugs of any kind. I stay away from **all** pharmaceutical medications. I do a tremendous amount of reading, as I refuse to subscribe to television in our home. I strive to keep our home a quiet and peaceful place to live.

In general, I am just very careful about how I subject my body.

I have been given a second chance on life with my history; **why jeopardize it.** With all of these practices that I instill with myself; I am very seldom sick in any way. I very seldom get colds and flu bugs on the seasonal changes. When a flu bug or cold does come to visit me, I credit my immune system as "reprogramming" itself to deal with the invader. Looking back in medical records, I was never even vaccinated as a baby or as a child due to my medical conditions at the time; and yet I made it to this day! I physically don't take too many chances for injury. No rock climbing, no jumping out of airplanes, no bungee jumping, no activity that might jeopardize my physical being.

My story is an excellent example of the tremendous innate power of the human body to adapt to the conditions at hand. My hope for you the reader is to realize and understand that ***anything is possible***! I want to pass on the desire and motivation, along with the realization to live life at a higher level. Have an awareness of all that is going on around you; not just sports teams, TV shows, and news. See the beauty in nature; see the beauty and grace in other people.

Experience things from a more enlightened point of view. Help rather than hinder, give aid rather than ignore, and reverberate peace rather than conflict; realize that *your* life is one of the greatest gifts.

This story is my **gift** to you……Enjoy everything !!

~Dr. Brad Schmidt

FACTS ABOUT ME

~ I am generally always *cold* when the temp falls below 70 degrees.

~ I have always found it difficult to gain weight no matter how much food I take consume.

~ I do not feel fatigue or pain from the left side of body from the waist down to my foot.

~ I have more body rotation to the left than I do to the right due to a rotatory scoliosis presentation.

~ The left side of my body starting from my waist down is significantly colder to the touch than the right.

~ I can only stand (balance) on my right leg and not my left leg.

~ I sometime collapse and fall to the ground because my left leg "gives out". I loose balance and fall if I don't brace myself on something.

~ Since I lost my hair to chemotherapy as a baby, it grew back thicker and grows at a faster rate. As an adult, I get a haircut every two weeks.

~I have one kidney significantly smaller in size and function than the other due to radiation treatment.

~ Due to the curvature of my scoliosis, my lowest rib on my left side almost touches my left hip.

FACTS ABOUT ME

~ My left leg is over an inch shorter than my right leg; therefore I make my own heel lifts for all my shoes.

~ I have what is called a step gait when I walk due to muscle instabilities on my left pelvis and left leg

~ I never think of myself as HANDICAPPED….my motto is "If you can do it…I can try to do it to!" I am "ok" not being able to perform some task…..I respect my limits.

~ I have had collectively over 250 x-rays in my lifetime.

~ I do not sleep for more than 5 hours at a time.

~ I still to this day, have a difficult time visiting a hospital even if it is to visit a friend who is the patient.

~ I have a high level of energy, always moving, always thinking.

~ I try to keep my complaining to a minimum.

~ I attempt to learn from *every* situation.

~ I never think in terms of failure…I think in results.

~ I tend to be singular rather than affiliated to a group.

~ I am less comfortable in crowds.

~ I read more books than I watch television.

~ I think about all my tasks and endeavors from the end; not the beginning.

~ I believe that you can figure out an individual by asking them to describe their 5 closest friends, name the last 5 books they read, and the last 5 movies they watched.

<u>AKNOWLEDGMENTS</u>

Upon the completion of the task of writing this book, I feel that I have finally unlocked all the rooms of my mind. I have shed light on to many of my darkest memories. To research and document my story has been a kind of therapy for my own understanding of all the events that have transpired. In regards to constructing and publishing this story, I would like to say a special thanks to Jim Langlais Esq., my confidant, my editor, and my attorney throughout this entire project. Special thanks, to Dr. Dirk Schroeder, editor and idealist. Dr. Schroeder assisted me in editing, web design, and marketing.

Another special consideration goes to my wife and best friend, Allison. Her support and input has been invaluable. She influenced me to keep assembling and writing the material to compile my story. She tolerated and respected my time to bring this project to reality. To my mother and father, Jackie and Charles, without you and your donation of interviews and documents, I could not have constructed the details that went into this book. As your son, I cannot ever say enough praise and thanks. This book is my gift to you both for all that you have endured with me.

I have so much respect for all the medical doctors, chiropractors, and nurses who played and continue to play an intricate role in my existence. Thank you to all of you for your tireless care, dedication, and donation of time. For in the end, I have made peace with my conflict and the damage it had rained on my body. I embrace it all, for cancer has made me who I am. I say a quiet 'thank you' to the powers that be, each time I open my eyes to wake in the morning.....I have one more 'gift' of new day on this earth.

In Peace,

Dr. Brad Schmidt